The Herbal
for Mother and Child

The Herbal
for Mother and Child

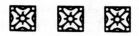

Anne McIntyre

ELEMENT
Shaftesbury, Dorset ● Boston, Massachusetts
Melbourne, Victoria

' Element Books Limited 1992
Text ' Anne McIntyre 1992

First published in the UK in 1992 by
Element Books Limited
Shaftesbury, Dorset SP7 8BP

Published in the USA in 1992 by
Element Books, Inc.
160 North Washington Street
Boston, MA 02114

Published in Australia in 1992 by
Element Books and distributed
by Penguin Australia Limited
487 Maroondah Highway, Ringwood,
Victoria 3134

Cover illustration by Rod Holt

Printed and bound in Great Britain by
Selwood Digital Printing

British Library Cataloguing in Publication
data available

Library of Congress Cataloging in Publication
data available

ISBN 1 852 30 244 5

CONTENTS

INTRODUCTION

This book is for our children. It is a manual to give advice to parents on caring for their off-spring from infancy throughout childhood, using the natural remedies around them – foods and medicinal herbs.

A child's health begins with the parents at the time of conception. Their health affects the sperm and egg – the stronger and fitter they are, the healthier the foetus. We pass on our genetic blueprint to our children, so it is vital that parents prepare positively for parenthood to give their offspring the best possible chance of optimum health and vitality. Our responsi-bilities to our children begin preconceptually, not simply once the baby is born, and they continue throughout pregnancy. The mother's good health throughout the gestation period will contribute significantly to a happy and problem-free pregnancy and a straightforward delivery of a healthy baby. From then on her dual responsibility changes – the new-born baby has his or her own separate needs and individual pattern of health, which develop alongside the mother's even though the baby is still very much dependent on her care.

Increasingly people are wanting to play a larger part in their own health care and that of their children. In the last twenty years the adoption of a healthy lifestyle has become a popular ideal for many, and evidence of this fills the media, bookshops and health-food shops. Most of us know very well that plenty of fresh air and exercise, rest and relaxation, and natural, wholesome foods are the prerequisites of good health and thereby our main source of preventative medicine. Parents are looking for still more information on how they can enhance their children's health and how they can treat their common ailments using safer and gentler alternatives to medicines such as antibiotics and steroids.

At the same time, many family doctors are becoming increasingly reluctant to prescribe drugs for these minor problems. As more information is available on self-help and on alternatives or supplements to orthodox medi-cal care, the relationship between patients and doctors is undergoing a metamorphosis. The rather authoritarian, father-like figure of the doctor is disappearing, while better informed and thereby more confident patients have greater freedom to choose the kind of treatment they or their family need. Patients and doctors are beginning to talk to each other on a more equal footing.

The emergence of complementary or holistic medicine has acted as a catalyst for this transformation. In the UK complementary practitioners, with their philosophy of self-help and the emphasis they place on enhancing our innate self-healing mechanisms, are increasing in numbers six times faster than doctors.[1] They exist alongside, not in compe-tition with, allopathic doctors. Now patients can choose what best suits their needs at the time from the therapies on offer. This greater independence means that there is no need to bother the doctor with every trivial or self-limiting problem nor to have to swallow unnecessary tablets, which can be kept for use in more serious illness. Even then, however, your self-help education will not be wasted. Much can be done to minimize the possible side-effects of drugs and to aid recovery – eat-ing special foods, taking extra vitamins and minerals, exercising in certain ways and so on. For example, it is now widely known that one of the consequences of taking antibiotics is the proliferation of *Candida albicans* (thrush) in the body. This can be prevented by taking natural live yoghurt or lacto-acidophilus tablets, garlic and olive oil, to help re-establish the beneficial bacterial population of the gut, upset by the antibiotic that allowed the fungal infection to flourish.

The most ancient of these increasingly popu-lar therapies is herbal medicine. In many instances herbs can provide a gentle and safe alternative or complement to drugs. They are compatible with the chemistry of the human body, which has adapted over thousands of years to assimilate them. The recognition of this is confirmed by the enormous resurgence of interest in all things herbal and the rediscov-ery of our medical roots. More and more parents are concerned to find safe, effective remedies for their babies and children, whose minor ailments often do not warrant the harsh-ness of powerful drugs. For example, atopic eczema can often be successfully treated by

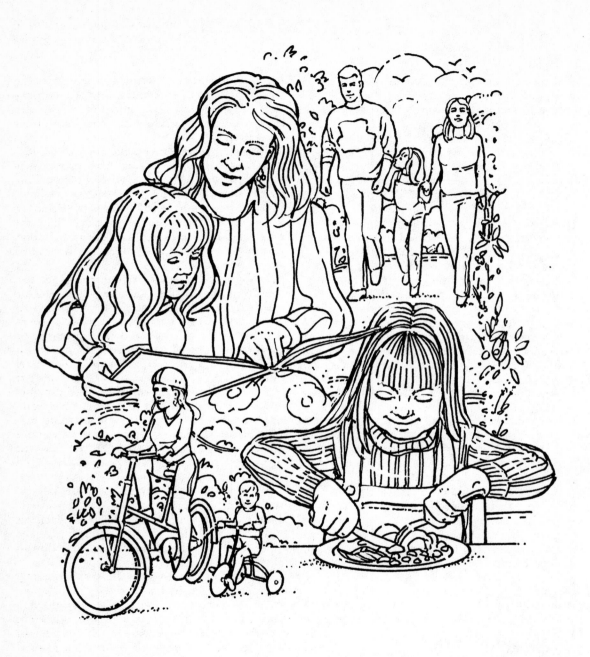

taking *evening primrose oil* and using *camomile cream* topically to replace hydrocortisone cream; while a milk-free diet may well augment this treatment as well as help to reduce over-frequent upper respiratory infections.

The new-born baby and the small child are the most vulnerable to the effects of drugs, because their eliminative systems are as yet not fully developed. A new-born baby may take several times longer to eliminate a drug from his or her tiny body than an adult, and so the infant can become overloaded with a drug that may affect an adult in only a very minor way.

Over the centuries we have developed an enormous wealth of information on the uses and efficacy of herbal medicines. Passed down

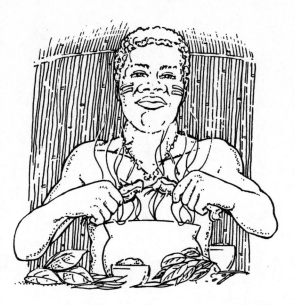

in this effort, and they propose cultural centres to improve and communicate knowledge of medicinal plants.[3]

Even developed, industrialized countries in which modern medicine is now well established, such as the UK, Europe, America and Japan, are looking towards herbs and their potential for health care. In all these countries a great deal of research is being carried out into medicinal plants. Papers are frequently published in leading medical journals on the therapeutic effects of herbs such as *ginseng, feverfew, evening primrose oil* and *garlic*, and of the numerous herbs that enhance the immune system, such as *echinacea* and *myrrh*,[4] with a view to their possible role in the treatment of AIDS.

This means that here in the West, we can combine the best of both worlds, blend the old with the new, turn to the folklore of ancient herbalism vindicated by the results of modern scientific research. In fact, there are many who are doing just this in a very professional way. In a way, modern herbal practitioners have replaced the 'wise old women', but they are well versed not only in the tradition and use of herbal medicine, but also in its biochemistry and pharmacology. In addition, they are well trained in conventional medical science, which they use against a background of a holistic approach to healing.

With the constant interchange of information and herbs between one tradition and another, the modern herbalist can also benefit from the wealth of knowledge from Chinese, Ayurvedic, Tibetan, Japanese, and North and South American Indian herbal traditions. The UK imports an enormous amount of herbs to augment those growing in our hedgerows. *Ginger, ginseng, echinacea, myrrh* and *cinnamon* are among the best known of the imported herbs, and they are indispensable to most herbal dispensaries. Herbal practitioners have set up all over the country, spreading the use of herbs with confidence, spurred on by our new Green consciousness, which reminds us constantly that this move towards a greater respect for nature must be urgently pursued if we are going to survive.

from generation to generation, it has stood the test of time until today, when the World Health Organization (WHO) informs us that 85 per cent of the world's population still use herbs as the main form of medical treatment, despite the introduction into many parts of the world of modern medical science, with its sophisticated chemical drugs and advanced technology.

And this is very fortunate, for in the late 1970s, after worldwide surveys by international health agencies, the Director General of WHO stated that, to achieve and maintain adequate health care for the world by the year 2000, we need to encourage and develop the use of traditional systems of medicine, for western orthodox medicine alone will not meet our medical needs.[2] In 1987 WHO stated that it had passed a resolution to urge countries to utilize traditional medical systems, and

to optimally use practitioners of traditional medicine; to initiate comprehensive programmes to investigate, cultivate and preserve medicinal plants; to assure the quality control of plant medicines by applying pharmaceutical standards and test methods; and to extend co-operation and sharing of skills between countries. WHO has ordered the Director General to mobilize funds to help

PART I

THE ROLE OF HERBS

CHAPTER 1

ENERGY FOR LIFE – LIVING SYSTEMS

The scientific approach to medicine views the human body as a combination of separate parts, almost as if each works individually without reference to each other or to the whole being. There are the different systems – the respiratory, digestive, urinary, reproductive and circulatory, for example; then there are the various organs – liver, heart, and kidneys and so forth; then there is the chemistry of the cells, the tissue fluid in which they are bathed and so on. The abundance of technical information, macroscopical and microscopical, on all these individual aspects of the body is fantastic. When we feel unwell or develop an ache or pain, we visit our doctor so that he can tell us which part is not functioning properly and prescribe something to take away the discomfort and soothe the pain – something that may well lull us into the false sense that all is well and that we have repaired the problem or cured the disease.

THE VITAL FORCE

We all know that we are far more than the machine this picture portrays. We do, of course, possess all the organs and systems so precisely described by medicine, but we have something over and above that; something that gives us the ability to grow, to change and repair ourselves, to adapt to new situations, to think creatively and to feel a whole range of emotions. We have *life*, which imbues our every cell. Each of us is born with an inherent healing wisdom that permeates our every dimension. It manifests itself in the amazing feats that we see daily, as the body continually protects, heals and regulates its organs and

functions. In the scientific world this is recognized as 'homoeostasis'. We maintain a steady state within our bodies, in our blood sugar levels, temperature, fluid balance, in the chemical composition of our blood and regularity of our respiration rate, despite the constantly present variables that could dangerously upset our equilibrium. Junk food, pollution in the atmosphere, contaminants in our water, stress and tension can all unbalance us, but despite these factors, we perennially demonstrate our powers of adaptation and self-healing.

These powers are central to the philosophy of holistic medicine. Within the different systems and therapies they are known as the life force, the vital force, Qi or prana. When a combination of pathogenic factors eventually manages to inhibit our homoeostatic mechanisms, our self-healing can become compromised and imbalances occur, and soon, if these are ignored, illness results. In the holistic approach it is recognized that when a specific symptom manifests itself, it is an expression of disharmony or disease within the whole being, not just the part apparently affected. To assist our self-healing and that of our children, we need to examine how a specific dysfunction in our body relates to the different aspects of ourselves and our lives – physical, mental, emotional and spiritual. Only then will we understand how to enhance our healing energies, and not hinder their efforts.

By observing ourselves, life within and without us, we will begin to see that we are subject to natural laws and forces. Our understanding of these will enable us to live our lives in accordance with them, not in violation of them, not only when we fall ill but also in our daily

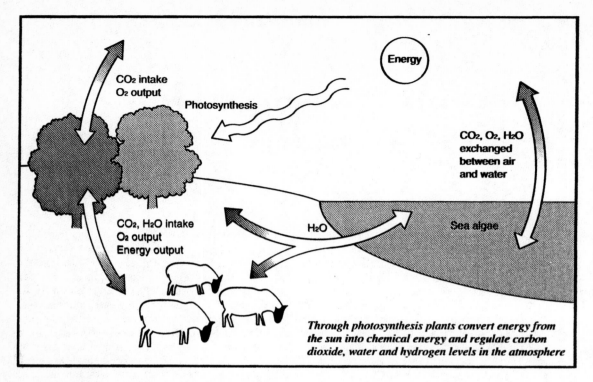

CO₂ intake
O₂ output

Photosynthesis

Energy

CO₂, O₂, H₂O
exchanged
between air
and water

CO₂, H₂O intake
O₂ output
Energy output

H₂O

Sea algae

Through photosynthesis plants convert energy from the sun into chemical energy and regulate carbon dioxide, water and hydrogen levels in the atmosphere

lives. Combining a healthy diet and lifestyle with the use of natural remedies to enhance the work of the vital force, will contribute to the maintenance of good health – ours and our children's.

HERBS AND ECOLOGY

Such observation will necessarily involve extending our awareness to perceive and understand our interconnectedness with the world outside us, our families, our community, our place in the world, the natural world around us and, ultimately, our relationship with the planet itself. We are the microcosm, the world around us the macrocosm. We cannot separate the two – what occurs in one is reflected in the other.

An increasing ecological awareness has been forced upon us by the crisis of increasing pollution and the destruction of the rain forests, which have led to such far-reaching global effects as the 'greenhouse effect', and they have also awakened a strong realization of our interconnectedness with the rest of the planet. Our lives and the life of everything in nature and everything on this planet, depend above all on

the sun. The life force, Qi, the energy for life, is derived from sunlight. It is solar energy.

Plants have the unique ability to store this solar energy. Through the process of photosynthesis they use the energy from the sun directly. Most plants contain a green colouring substance, chlorophyll, which enables them to use the sun's energy to make sugars by taking in water and carbon dioxide from their environment. From sunlight, carbon dioxide and water they also synthesize proteins, enzymes, hormonal substances and oils. Although these substances are produced for the plants' own homoeostasis, they are of great value to humans. From the soil plants take up elements, such as phosphorus, nitrogen and potassium, which provide us with vital nutrients.

Not only do we all depend on these substances for our food (and the animals we eat have also depended on them), but we also depend upon the oxygen that plants give out while making their food. Thus plants, by trapping the sun's energy through photosynthesis, enable this energy to be accessible to every inhabitant of the earth. It is this solar energy which provides energy for us, from the minutest biochemical reaction to the contraction of

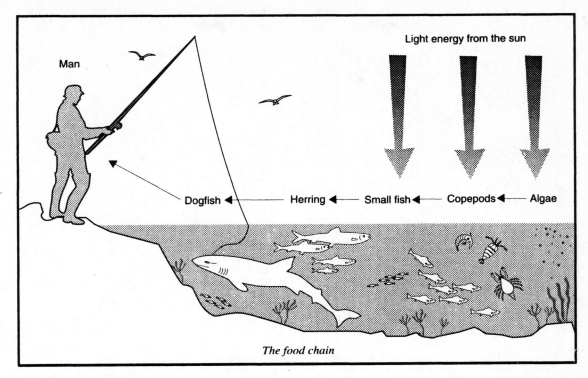

Man

Light energy from the sun

Dogfish ← Herring ← Small fish ← Copepods ← Algae

The food chain

large muscles. And yet plants do still more than this. In addition to producing oxygen they also regulate the carbon dioxide, water and hydrogen levels in the atmosphere, thus having a direct impact on the temperature of the earth and the atmosphere. The destruction of the rain forests has raised carbon dioxide levels, which contributes to global warming and the melting of the ice caps. It is clear that we humans do not exist in isolation. The constant interaction between us and the environment, our ecology, can be illustrated easily by the food chain (see Figure above).

The element carbon is also vital for the function of protoplasm in every cell, plant, animal and human alike (see Figure on page 16).

Our relationship with plants is symbiotic. Plants provide us with food and drink, shelter, raw materials, such as wood, cotton, paper, oils, dyes and perfumes, and they rely on us and on the animal world for carbon dioxide and pollination, and on bacteria in the soil to break down dead remains and return their constituents to the cycle of life in the earth and the atmosphere.

As we have moved away from using the basic raw materials provided by the earth to a highly technological society, capable of producing an enormous range of synthetic chemicals, we have upset this natural symbiotic relationship. As the results of this become increasingly evident, the reverence and respect for plant life that we had in former times has begun to reassert itself. Green issues have come to the fore, and plants and herbs are becoming apparent in many areas of modern life – herbal cosmetics and shampoos, teas and foods, fabrics and wallpapers, the advertising world, and books galore.

Having said this, we may hardly be surprised at the central role that medicinal herbs have held in our lives throughout history. The use of herbs reflects the interdependence of man and plants, and their role in healing as medicines reflects holism in its wider aspects. Our harmonious relationship with nature, enlivened by the same vital force, is illustrated by the ability of the herbal world to provide us with the perfect medicines for so many of our ills – as will be shown throughout this book.

By utilizing the energy and healing constituents contained in herbs to redress the imbalances that contribute to our ill-health, we can restore harmony within ourselves and with our environment. By taking herbs into our bodies to restore health and vitality, we can

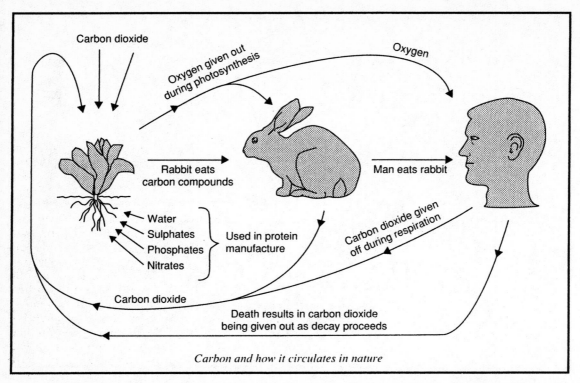

Carbon dioxide

Oxygen given out during photosynthesis

Oxygen

Rabbit eats carbon compounds

Man eats rabbit

Water
Sulphates
Phosphates
Nitrates

Used in protein manufacture

Carbon dioxide given off during respiration

Carbon dioxide

Death results in carbon dioxide being given out as decay proceeds

Carbon and how it circulates in nature

offer more to the world around us. Since we cannot separate ourselves, our health and our healing from our ecology, by healing ourselves we may perhaps also help to heal our planet. Health depends not only on the right environment and the right foods, but also on our thoughts, feelings, aspirations and our relationship to ourselves, others and the world around us. Herbs work at a physiological level, but through their influence not only on the body but also on the nervous system, they can help to establish a basis of physical and mental health as a springboard to life. By balancing our physical functions and enhancing our vital energy, we have a greater possibility of integrating all the different aspects of our being: emotional, mental and spiritual.

CHAPTER 2

UNDERSTANDING HERBS

THE HERBAL APPROACH TO HEALING

A tradition of herbal medicine and the veneration of the medicinal values of wild plants are common to cultures all over the world; in fact, there are almost no peoples studied by anthropologists who have not used plants as medicines as part of their culture.[1] Herbalism is the most ancient form of medicine known to man, and its present recognition is nothing new; it is simply an echo, fast becoming a reverberating sound, of the past.

Certainly the West's growing interest in herbal medicine may involve much rediscovery of our medical roots, but herbal traditions in other parts of the world – such as China, Tibet and India – are alive and well as they have been for thousands of years. Their philosophies and systems have remained almost intact to this day and have much to teach us who have long forgotten such wisdom and now thirst for it. Basic to these traditions is the understanding that health is derived from a balance of natural forces in the body, and illness occurs when this balance is disturbed; that the body has an inherent ability to regulate and heal itself, which herbal medicines have the ability to support and enhance. Here in the West we have been re-evaluating our understanding of *health*. It does not just mean absence of symptoms. It is, in the words of the World Health Organization: 'The condition of perfect bodily, spiritual and social well-being and not solely the absence of illness and injury.'

So, health depends on the harmony of body, mind and spirit, and any imbalance or illness needs to be seen in relation to the patient as a whole, in the context of the patient's life – inner and outer. As Plato wrote in *The Republic*:

> The cure of the part should not be attempted without the treatment of the whole. No attempt should be made to cure the body without the soul and if the head and body are to be healthy, you must begin by curing the mind.

With this in mind, herbs can be prescribed not solely to be directed to the area of disturbance to diminish the symptoms, but to attend to the deeper causes of imbalance. In the Indian medicine traditions of North and South America, herbs have been revered for their ability to cure not only diseases of the body, but also imbalances in the realms of emotion, mind and spirit. Herbs have been an inextricable part of their religion or mythology and were used in ceremonies and rituals. Disease is seen to be due either to human, supernatural or natural causes, and the medicine man or woman is called upon to administer herbs for anything from wounds and broken bones to unfulfilled dreams, spirit intrusion and soul loss.[2] Small wonder that to these people, plants have been represented as symbols of the magic and power of nature, which they worshipped and glorified.

PLANTS AND DRUGS

The beneficial effect of medicinal plants can be confirmed to any doubting Thomas when one considers that the origins of many modern medicines lie in herbs. They have been the source of a wide range of potent medicines, and may form the basis of many effective and widely used drugs that are still employed today. Quinine, a derivative of *cinchona* (or *Peruvian bark*) is the basis of anti-malarial drugs still prescribed in modern surgeries; *ipecacuanha* is still used as an emetic; atropine, codeine, digoxin, digitoxin, morphine and ephedrine are all plant-derived drugs of unquestionable value found in modern pharmacological textbooks and dispensaries. Other herbs have been employed as a model for synthesis of similar substances manufactured in laboratories. The *white willow (Salix alba)* provided salicylic acid which has been replaced by the synthetic drug aspirin; the *foxglove* provided us with the model for digoxin. The list goes on and on.

Much of the modern medical disdain for the old-fashioned herbal remedies that are becoming popular now has its roots in a former kind of ethnic arrogance on the part of the medical establishment that prevented scientists from paying serious attention or ascribing any virtue to the herbal or medical knowledge of peoples such as the 'savages' of North and South America. The 'superstitious' rites accompanying their healing practices were repellent to the 'educated', logical brains of the first explorers and settlers.[3] Once they had recognized the value of the Indians' herbal lore, they incorporated much of it into their own medicine. It was later adopted by American 'folk medicine' of the eighteenth and nineteenth centuries. Only at this point did some of the amazing Indian discoveries begin to attract the well-deserved attention of medical scientists and thereby open up new frontiers in medical history.

Coca was the 'divine plant' of the Incas, and South American Indians chew the leaves to this day, to give them strength and endurance on journeys and to conquer hunger and pain. It is said to have been used as an anaesthetic in pre-Columbian trephination (skull surgery). Coca was largely ignored by medical scientists until the nineteenth century, but its main active alkaloid, cocaine, was isolated in 1806, and in 1884 Carl Koller discovered its value as a local anaesthetic. Many other discoveries have their origins in 'savage' medicine. Frederick Banting had to attribute much of the credit for his discovery of insulin to the knowledge of the Indians, while researchers were led to the contraceptive pill by analysing the medicinal herbs that Indians used to suppress ovulation.

Scientists, with their mechanistic approach, have tended to view medicinal plants as a source of active ingredients, analysing the chemicals under the microscope and assessing their pharmacological effects in the body only in terms of their biochemistry. It is, of course, true that herbal preparations do operate at the level of biochemical reactions in the body, but their history and mythology have shown us that they are capable of far more. They do provide us with a wealth of valuable chemicals, but their healing powers go beyond the physical to the realm of the vital force, that invisible life energy that animates us on every level of existence, physical, emotional, mental and spiritual. Through their initial action in the

physical body, the herbs enhance the healing action of this vital force, and as they do this they may also heal our hearts and minds as they help to restore harmony to an integrated whole being. Perhaps this idea is what the Indians interpreted in their own way, when using herbs for 'soul loss' and 'unfulfilled dreams'.

THE WHOLE PLANT

With the development of science and chemistry came the introduction into medicine of single, active components, which were isolated from plants to replace the use of whole plant medicines. As these substances began to be manufactured synthetically, herbs that had been revered for centuries were being declared old-fashioned and obsolete. Doctors and pharmacologists believed that if the chemical formula of a man-made product were similar to that of one from nature, it would be assimilated just as easily by our bodies.

This view, however, does not coincide with the principles of medical herbalists, and through many unfortunate and tragic incidents, it is becoming clear that the isolation and synthesis of active components based on plant medicines, and many modern inventions in the drug world besides, have produced an array of unforeseen, unpleasant and sometimes serious side-effects. The plant-derived drugs already mentioned – atropine, morphine, ephedrine and digoxin – are effective but extremely potent as isolated, active constituents, and they have to be used with great caution. People are looking for safer alternatives, gentler, perhaps slower-acting, but without side-effects.

Recently we have seen that even aspirin, that household name and derivative of natural plant substances, has not stood the test of time. It has been declared unsafe for children, and in 1986 all children's aspirin-based drugs were withdrawn from the market because aspirin was implicated in its association with Reye's syndrome in children, as a sequel to other childhood diseases, causing damage to the kidneys and the brain.

The modern herbalist still advocates the use of the whole plant, not isolated, active constituents, as a gentler and safer form of treatment. Two main types of substances are found in medicinal herbs, both of which have an equally important role to play therapeutically. The primary healing agents are the active constituents, which seized the imagination of the early chemists and which have developed into modern medical drugs. Then there are other, apparently secondary and less important agents, whose actual value should not be overlooked. They play an essential role in determining how effective the primary healing agents will be, by rendering the body more or less receptive to their powers. Some of these 'synergistic' substances will make the active constituents more assimilable and readily available in the body, while others will buffer the action of other potent plant chemicals, thus preventing any possible side-effects. It is the natural combination of both types of plant substances that determines the healing power and safety of the remedy.

THE CHEMISTRY OF HERBS

Because we have always eaten plants, our bodies have adapted over thousands of years to respond to plant medicines in a way they never can to man-made drugs. Herbs are actually very much like foods, and the dividing line between them is very thin. By definition a herb is any plant that has a therapeutic action on the body, and this includes most of the fruit and vegetable kingdom. For example, *raspberries* are full of vitamins and minerals; in addition to their delicious taste, they have long been used for throat and chest problems, and the whole plant is well known for a variety of uses during pregnancy and childbirth.

Garlic and *onions* are excellent health-promoting and medicinal foods. They contain sulphur, germanium and selenium, important trace elements and especially valuable in supporting the immune system. Grains, nuts and seeds contain antibiotic-resistant factors, which increase natural resistance to disease. They also contain auxones, which help to produce vitamins in the body and are involved in the rejuvenation of cells, thereby slowing the ageing process. *Carrots* contain vitamin A precursors (beta carotene) and vitamin C, which are useful for stubborn skin disorders and chronic eye infections, and for increasing the body's resistance and tolerance to poisons and infections. They are also used beneficially for ailments of the urinary tract.

As well as a wide variety of minerals, vitamins and trace elements, herbs contain a variety of different types of substances known to have specific therapeutic actions in the body. The more widely investigated of these are described below.

Volatile Oils

Most of us are familiar with herbs that contain high concentrations of volatile oils – the highly scented culinary herbs such as *rosemary, oregano, thyme, sage, mint, fennel* and *dill* which lend that wonderful aroma and taste to cooking all over the world. While we are enjoying pasta with *fresh basil*, roast lamb with *mint* sauce and steamed fish with *dill* or *parsley* sauce, we are also administering to ourselves in the simplest way imaginable, valuable therapeutic herbs with volatile oils.

Volatile or essential oils are composed of a wide variety of chemical compounds, and the many combinations of these produce the wonderful variation in their aromas and therapeutic effects. Up to fifty different ingredients have been identified in some oils. As the constituents vary, so do the actions of the herbs containing them. All volatile oils have antiseptic and antibiotic properties, which enhance the action of the immune system in warding off bacterial, viral or fungal invasion and infection. Many oils have anti-inflammatory and anti-spasmodic properties: those in *camomile*, for example, are useful in the relief of inflamed, irritated conditions and colicky pain; *dill* is the active therapeutic agent in gripe water, which is used for colic in babies. Some oils – *thyme* and *hyssop*, for example – have an expectorant action, hastening the expulsion of mucus from the chest. Other oils are diuretic and are useful where there is water retention or urinary infection. Some oils act as tonics, enhancing the function of the stomach, intestines, gall-bladder and liver. Others stimulate the heart and circulation.

Volatile oils can be ingested in different ways – they can be taken in foods and drinks, they can be rubbed on to the skin or inhaled. Their actions are felt throughout the digestive system, urinary system, and the respiratory system, as well as affecting sweat, salivary, vaginal and lachrimal (from the eye) secretions. In the case of a lactating mother, the oils are passed to the baby through the breast milk.

Fennel, dill or *camomile* tea drunk by a lactating mother can soothe baby's colic and induce relaxing sleep.

Since the time of the ancient Egyptians we have made use of the therapeutic properties of volatile oils. The art of employing the aromas of these oils, now known as aromatherapy, also has a long tradition in the Far East. When we breathe in the scent of herbs containing a high proportion of volatile oils, we stimulate certain nerve endings situated in the upper part of the nose, and these carry nerve impulses or messages to the brain, especially the limbic system, the area that relates to certain of our mental or emotional states. When they are rubbed on the skin, the oils stimulate nerve endings in the skin, and messages are relayed to the underlying tissues, muscles, blood and lymphatic vessels, and also, via the nervous system, to the pituitary gland, the gland that regulates the action of all other endocrine glands, including the adrenal glands. These effects make aromatherapy of enormous benefit in relieving stress and enhancing relaxation. *Rose* oil is especially useful in women's problems, for alleviating tension and anxiety and symptoms related to the reproductive system, such as problems around the menstrual cycle, anxiety about childbirth, sexual difficulties or postnatal depression. *Camomile* oil diluted and added to bath water is wonderful for fractious children (and mothers!) at the end of the day; it will encourage deep and relaxing sleep for both.

Tannins

The predominant therapeutic action of tannins is astringent, and it is brought about by their ability to bind albumin, a protein in the skin and mucous membranes, to form a tight, insoluble, protective layer that is resistant to disease. On the skin or in the delicate linings of the mouth, the respiratory, digestive, urinary and reproductive systems, tannins can separate bacteria that threaten to invade the body from their source of nutrition. Tannins also have a healing action, protecting these areas from irritation while at the same time reducing inflammation. Tannins occur widely in nature, and they are the predominant therapeutic constituents in herbs such as *witch hazel, shepherd's purse, tormentil* and *oak bark*. They are used as mouth washes for infected and bleeding gums, gargles for sore throats, medicines for catarrh, inflammation of the digestive tract and diarrhoea, compresses to heal abrasions and wounds, and in hot water to bathe haemorrhoids and inflamed skin conditions.

Bitters

Many herbal remedies contain chemicals with a bitter taste. These substances exert their medicinal action mainly in the digestive tract, where they promote the secretion of digestive juices in the stomach and intestines and the flow of bile in the liver. Bitter herbs are prescribed for loss of appetite, heartburn, weak and sluggish digestion, gastritis, anaemia, nervous exhaustion and to aid convalescence after influenza or other, more debilitating, illness. Many bitter herbs have other qualities – some are relaxant and sedative, others are anti-inflammatory; some exert a beneficial action on the immune system, acting as natural antibiotics and anti-neoplastic (anti-tumour) remedies. Well-known 'bitter tonics' include *dandelion, centaury, chicory* and *dock root, wormwood* and *gentian*. Their therapeutic action begins in the mouth and so, for good effect, despite many people's distaste for bitters, must be tasted.

Mucilage

Mucilage is a sugary, gel-like substance that is found widely in plants. It has the ability to draw water to it, and when it is added to water it swells up to form a viscous fluid. Because of this, plants containing mucilage can have a mild laxative effect because they loosen the bowel contents by absorbing water into the bowel. *Psyllium* seeds do just this. One or two teaspoons of seeds left to soak in a cup of cold water for 30 minutes can be taken morning and night to relieve constipation, and they are perfectly safe for use in pregnancy and for children.

Alkaloids

Alkaloids are compounds which all contain nitrogen, and they tend to have potent effects, often being toxic in large amounts. They are frequently found in herbs whose use is restricted to qualified medical herbalists and doctors, and they are often unsuitable for home use in herbal teas. They vary widely in their components and actions in the body, but they often affect the nervous system in particular. They include morphine, from the *opium poppy*, atropine, which is found in *deadly nightshade*, caffeine and theobromide, which occur in *coffee, black tea* and *cocoa,* and nicotine, which is, of course, found in *tobacco.* Alkaloids are also present in small, non-toxic amounts in other herbs, where they act as catalysts to other healing agents without being involved themselves – for example, pyrrolizioline alkaloids in *comfrey* and *coltsfoot.*

Cardiac Glycosides

These are substances containing a sugar combined with a cardio-active, non-sugar component. They are present in *broom, foxglove, lily-of-the-valley, squills* and *wallflowers.* They have a particular affinity to the heart, supporting a weak heart and stabilizing the function of the heart muscle. They are, therefore, used for heart failure and arrhythmias to produce more coordinated and efficient contractions of the heart muscle and an increase in muscle power. Digoxin is the cardiac glycoside derived from *foxglove*, which is famous among allopathic doctors, but modern herbalists prefer to use *lily-of-the-valley*, because it has a gentler action as its cardiac glycosides are released more slowly and excreted more easily, thus avoiding toxic accumulation in the body.

Flavonoids

Flavonoids or flavonoid glycosides occur commonly in plants. They impart a yellow/orange colour, as in *cowslips* and *oranges*, and have a sweet or bitter taste. Most flavonoids have a diuretic action – *buchu* and *parsley*, for example – some such as *liquorice* are antispasmodic and anti-inflammatory, and others are antiseptic. Some are well-known as bioflavonoids, which occur in vitamin C-rich plants such as *blackcurrants* and *citrus fruits* and which act synergistically with ascorbic acid to enhance the body's ability to metabolize it. Bioflavonoids also act to strengthen and heal peripheral blood vessel walls and are used to treat a variety of vascular problems, such as bruising, bleeding (nose-bleeds, for instance) as well as high blood pressure.

Saponins

Saponins are glycosides that form a soap-like lather when they are mixed with water. *Soapwort (Saponaria officinalis)*, which contains a high proportion of saponins, was used in the past to manufacture soap. Saponins emulsify oils and are able to dissolve red blood cells, even when used in small amounts, and so they should never be injected directly into the bloodstream. Taken orally, however, they are hardly absorbed at all through an intact intestinal wall but instead help to promote digestion and absorption of many other substances, such as calcium and silicon. Saponins have a wide variety of actions. Some have a diuretic action, as in *horsetail* and *asparagus*; others have an expectorant effect, as in *cowslips* and *mullein* and some, such as those in *horse-chestnut*, exert a beneficial effect on blood vessel walls, reducing fragility and oedema by making the vein wall less permeable.

The most interesting saponins are the steroidal ones, which are similar in structure to human hormones secreted by the testes, ovaries and adrenal glands. Some steroidal saponins resemble cholesterol, cortisone, oestrogen, progesterone and vitamin D, while others, known as tri-terpenoid saponins, have the ability to regulate the steroidal hormonal activity in the body and to counter the effect of stress. Remedies containing these hormone-regulating properties are known as adaptogens, the most famous of which is *ginseng (Panax ginseng)*. Other adaptogenic herbs include *liquorice, false unicorn root, blue* and *black cohosh, squaw vine, wild yam* and *fenugreek.* Some of these herbs such as *wild yam* and *liquorice*, also exert an anti-inflammatory action.

Anthraquinones

These glycosides have a yellow colour that has often been used for producing commercial dyes. When taken internally, they stimulate the wall of the large intestine and thereby increase the force of muscular contraction, producing a laxative effect. They are found in herbs such as *senna, aloes, dock, cascara* and *alder*, and can sometimes cause griping in the bowel and so are better when combined with herbs such as *ginger* or *fennel*. They should never be used over a long period of time because they can reduce the normal bowel reflexes and cause habituation.

CHAPTER 3

PREPARATION OF HERBS

There are many ways in which we can prepare herbs to affect us beneficially. As long as they interact with our body chemistry in one way or another, they will exert their influence.

The basic ways of preparing herbs and of extracting their therapeutic properties for home use are old and traditional and have hardly changed since the time of the ancient Egyptians. The most natural and obvious way to take herbs into our systems is, of course, to eat them, which most of us, knowingly or not, do every day – salads with *parsley*, fish with *dill*, new potatoes with fresh *mint*, casseroles with *bay leaves*, pizza with *marjoram*, wine cups with *borage flowers*. As the foods are absorbed from the digestive tract, so the therapeutic constituents of the herbs enter the bloodstream, and from there can circulate throughout the body. Most of our traditional culinary herbs contain high proportions of volatile oils with their anti-microbial actions, and these would have been vital for health as well as for enhancing culinary skills in the days before refrigerators when meat hung in the market place for hours or even days.

The skin is highly absorbent, and a simple way to use herbs beneficially is to apply them in one way or another to the skin, where tiny blood capillaries under the surface will take their constituents into the bloodstream and thence through the body. Dilute essential oils can be rubbed into the skin, alcoholic rubbing lotions can be applied, as can ointments and creams, compresses and poultices, or leaves or flowers picked directly from the garden or country lane can be used to relieve a nettle sting, soothe a minor burn or staunch bleeding from a cut or graze.

The conjunctiva of the eye will also absorb herbal extracts, as anyone who has used a *camomile* eye bath or a *marigold* compress to relieve sore and inflamed eyes will have realized. The nose and nerve endings lying in it will provide another therapeutic pathway, as in the aromatherapy tradition. By inhalation, the messages from the herbs are carried directly to the brain, and are also taken into the lungs where they are absorbed with oxygen into the bloodstream and circulated throughout the system.

PREPARATION FOR INTERNAL USE

Infusions

Infusions are made in much the same way as an ordinary cup of tea, and are made from the soft parts of plants – leaves, stems and flowers.

Standard Infusion

Add 1oz (25g) of dried herb (or 2oz (50g) if fresh) to 1 pint (600ml) of boiling water, or a teaspoon per cup. This can, however, vary according to taste – it is important that it is palatable if you are to drink it regularly. Place the herbs in a warmed pot, pour on boiling water and cover immediately to prevent the valuable oils from escaping into the atmosphere. Leave to infuse for 10–15 minutes and then strain. The infusion can be drunk immediately or stored in an airtight container for up to two days in a refrigerator.

Some herbs need to be made up as cold infusions, because their therapeutic components

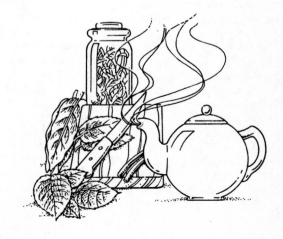

are likely to be destroyed by high temperatures. These include herbs that have a high proportion of mucilage such as *marshmallow root* and *comfrey*. They are prepared in the same way, but with cold water and left to infuse for 10–12 hours.

Dosage for Infusions

Infusions are normally taken by the cupful, three times daily in chronic problems and more frequently in acute illness. Half or quarter doses are suitable for children and babies.

Contrary to expectation, many medicinal herbs are found by our pampered palates to taste unpleasant, accustomed as we are to sugary and savoury tastes. Although the bitters in some plants need to be tasted to be efficacious, the bitter taste is not something most of us relish. However, it is possible to combine several herbs in an infusion, so that herbs such as *peppermint, lemon balm, lemon verbena* and *lavender* can disguise other, less palatable, herbs while not reducing their effect. Infusions can also be flavoured with *liquorice* or *aniseed* and sweetened with honey, which is a particularly useful means of enticing children to take them.

When we drink infusions we are following a tradition that had largely died out in the UK until recently but that has survived until the present in most other European countries. In France, Spain, Italy and Greece, tisanes of *lemon balm, camomile, elderflower, peppermint* and *limeflowers* have been taken as part of daily life. Bitter aperitifs are taken before a meal to stimulate the flow of digestive juices; digestifs are taken afterwards to ease digestion and settle the stomach.

Infusions are usually taken hot, particularly in the treatment of fevers, colds and catarrh, or lukewarm or cold for problems associated with the kidneys and urinary tract, such as kidney infections, cystitis, urethritis and bed-wetting in children.

Herbal tea bags are sold in all health food shops and many supermarkets, and usually comprise the more aromatic, pleasant-tasting herbs, such as *mint, camomile, fennel,* or delicious and exotic combinations of herbs and fruits. You can, of course, buy your chosen herbs loose (see Appendix 4 for a list of suppliers) and improvise your own mixtures to suit your or your children's taste and according to the effects you require.

Decoctions

The hard, woody parts of plants have tough cell walls, which need greater heat to break them down so that they release their ingredients into the water. Bark, seeds, roots, rhizomes and nuts all need to be prepared as decoctions. To make their constituents more accessible to water break them up into small pieces in a pestle and mortar, chop them with a knife if they are fresh, or smash with a hammer if they are very hard. It is often simpler to buy them ready powdered, although you can powder them yourself in a coffee grinder.

Standard Decoction

Use the same proportions of herb to water as for an infusion but add a little more water to make up for slight losses during preparation. Place the herbs in a stainless steel or enamelled saucepan (do not use aluminium as some plant constituents interact with this soft metal), and cover them with cold water. Bring to the boil, *cover* and simmer gently for 10–15 minutes. Strain and drink in the same dosage as an infusion.

Syrups

Syrups are a wonderful way in which to prescribe herbs for children, and they can be used to mask the taste of more unpleasant-tasting herbs.

Making Syrups

Pour 1 pint (600ml) of boiling water over 2½lb (1.25kg) of soft brown sugar and stir over a gentle heat until all the sugar has dissolved and the solution comes to the boil. If you have herbal tinctures, you can mix one part tincture to three parts syrup, and this will keep indefinitely.

If you have made an infusion or decoction, mix ¾lb (325g) sugar into 1 pint (600ml) of the liquid and heat until the sugar has dissolved. This should be kept in a cool place, preferably in a refrigerator. Alternatively, make an infusion or a decoction, strain it, weigh it and add to it a quarter of its weight of honey. Heat the liquid slowly and stir it until it begins to thicken, skimming off any scum that forms on the surface.

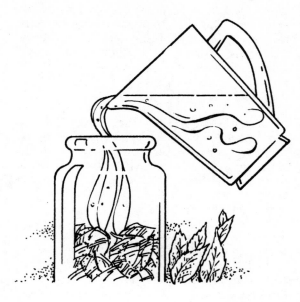

Dosage for Syrups

This depends on how it is prepared, but generally for children about a dessertspoonful should be taken three or four times daily.

Honey can also be used to persuade small children to take herbal remedies. Fresh powdered or dried herbs can be infused in runny honey and given on the spoon. You can also give essential oils in honey – one drop per teaspoon of honey.

Tinctures

Tinctures are more concentrated extracts of herbs that use a mixture of water and alcohol to extract the chemical constituents of the plant and to act as a preservative. When herbalists or manufacturers prepare tinctures, reference is made to a herbal pharmacopoeia, which lays down the correct ratio of water and alcohol to plant matter. This varies from one plant to another according to the therapeutic ingredients that need to be extracted. It can range

from 25 per cent alcohol for simple glycosides and tannins to 90 per cent alcohol for resins and gums.

Making Tinctures

The required herb can be used fresh or dried, either finely chopped or powdered. Place the herb in a large jar and pour the alcohol and water solution over it. When you use dried herbs, the standard preparation is one part herb to five parts fluid. Fresh plants are used in a ratio of one part herb to two parts fluid.

For example, to make $1\frac{3}{4}$ pints (1 litre) of *camomile* tincture, take 7oz (200g) of dried flowers and pour over $1\frac{3}{4}$ pints (1 litre) of fluid. *Camomile* requires a 45 per cent alcohol solution, and brandy or vodka would be perfectly adequate for home use (60–70 per cent proof is approximately equal to 45 per cent alcohol). Pour $1\frac{3}{4}$ pints (1 litre) of brandy or vodka over the herb, place an airtight lid on the jar and leave to macerate away from direct sunlight for no less than two weeks, shaking the jar well once or twice daily. After this, the mixture will be ready to press through a muslin bag, squeezing as much of the fluid as possible from the herb so as to waste as little as possible. You can use a simple wine-press to facilitate the process. Discard the herb once the fluid has been squeezed out – it makes very good compost – transfer the tincture to a dark bottle and store it in a cool place.

Some tinctures can be made using neat cider vinegar, when the acetic acid acts as a solvent and preservative. Some herbal vinegars, with *tarragon*, *garlic* or *rosemary*, are used in the kitchen, while *raspberry* vinegar is commonly used for coughs and sore throats and for children's respiratory ailments.

You can also make glycerol-based tinctures. Glycerol has a sweet, syrup-like taste, which makes it excellent for children and squeamish adults. Equal parts of water and glycerol should be poured over dried herbs, but 80 per cent glycerol is necessary for the more watery, fresh herbs such as *borage* and *comfrey* to prevent deterioration and infection. The process is otherwise the same as for alcoholic tinctures. *Peppermint*, *catmint*, *elderflowers*, *red clover*, *nettles*, *comfrey* and *marshmallow* are well suited to this method.

Dosage for Tinctures

Because they are concentrated, only small amounts need to be taken at a time at regular intervals through the day. The standard adult dose is 1 teaspoonful, and anything from 10 drops to ½ a teaspoonful for children, taken three times daily. In acute illness the dosage could be doubled. Tinctures can be taken undiluted or in a little water, children's juices or herbal teas. They can also be added to bath water, mixed with water to make compresses or in a base to make ointments or creams.

Tinctures require a little more time to make than do infusions or decoctions, but they have several advantages. They are easy to store, and they keep almost indefinitely (although they are probably best used within two years).. In addition, they do not suffer from being kept in cold, damp conditions.

Tablets and Capsules

Many herbs can be bought in tablet or capsule form from herb suppliers or health food shops, and this is a more convenient way of taking herbs.

Making Capsules

The more conscientious of you can make them up at home using powdered herbs. Gelatine capsules can be filled with mixtures of the appropriate herbs using a capsule maker (for Addresses, see Appendix 1), which enables you to make up a large quantity at a time. There are two main capsule sizes, 0 and 00. Size 0 holds approximately 0.35g of powder, so that three capsules (one or two for children) are needed three times daily to achieve the standard dose. Size 00 hold about 0.5g of powder, so two capsules (one for children) need to be taken three times daily.

When herbs are taken in pill or capsule form they bypass the taste buds on the tongue. Although this might be seen as a definite advantage in many cases, there are some herbs that ideally should not be taken in this way; this is particularly true of the bitter remedies taken for the liver and digestive tract, which, for maximum therapeutic benefit, need to be tasted to trigger reflexes in the rest of the digestive system.

Suppositories

The advantage of using suppositories to insert into the rectum is that the herbal remedy can be absorbed directly into the bloodstream through the mucosa of the rectum. This enables local and systemic problems to be treated quickly and simply, obviating the more laborious process of taking herbs by mouth to travel the distance of the alimentary canal before being absorbed into the system.

Making Suppositories

An easy way to prepare a suppository at home is to add finely powdered, dried herb to a base of melted cocoa butter, place it into a mould improvised to the required shape from aluminium foil, allow it to cool and store in the fridge. It is best to make a row of suppositories in the foil all at once.

PREPARATION FOR EXTERNAL USE

Many herbal constituents are absorbed readily through the skin, and these various preparations are designed to enhance this pathway into the body.

Herbal Baths

A wonderfully luxurious and relaxing way to take herbal medicines is in a fragrant hot bath. It is also a very easy way to give remedies to babies and children.

Preparing a Herbal Bath

There are various ways to add herbs to a bath: you can add a couple of drops of essential oil to the water (use only dilute oils for babies and children); you can hang a muslin bag with fresh (or dried) aromatic herbs straight from the garden under the hot tap; or you can add a pint (600ml) of strong herbal infusion to the water and then soak in the bath for 10–30 minutes.

When they are used in these ways, the essential oils from the plants are taken in through the pores of the skin, which are opened up by the warmth of the water. The oils are also carried on the steam into the atmosphere of your bathroom, to be inhaled via the nose and mouth into the lungs and thence into the bloodstream. From the nose the oils send messages via nerve receptors to the brain. The remedies are assimilated quickly and directly, bypassing the lengthy process of digestion that is necessary when remedies are taken by mouth. They are especially useful for relaxing and soothing the nervous system and easing mental and emotional strain. *Lavender* and *camomile* are wonderfully relaxing and beautifully fragrant, and will ease away anxiety and tension, helping to ensure a restful sleep. *Camomile* can be used for fractious children, especially if they are a little under the weather, for not only does it have antibiotic qualities but it also helps to induce sleep, nature's best way of warding off children's illness and aiding recovery. *Rosemary* baths, while also relaxing, are probably more suitable in the morning, as *rosemary* has a stimulating edge, sending blood to the brain, enhancing alertness and concentration. *Limeflower* baths are commonly used in France to help children sleep.

Hand and Foot Baths

Mustard foot baths are a traditional remedy for all afflictions of cold and damp climates, from colds and influenza to poor circulation and arthritis.

The ancient tradition of hand and foot baths has been resurrected to great effect by the French herbalist, Maurice Messegue, who has written several books on herbal therapy based simply on using this form of treatment. He recommends foot baths for eight minutes in the evening and hand baths for eight minutes in the morning. The hands and feet are very sensitive areas of the skin, full of nerve endings, and, despite some thickening of the skin from much use, the constituents pass easily from the skin into the body. Hand and foot baths are excellent ways of treating babies and children, who are required to keep still for only half the time recommended for adults – that is, four minutes each morning and evening.

Ointments and Creams

Ointments and creams can be used to treat skin problems such as eczema, but they will also reach less superficial ills, such as varicose veins and aching or inflamed joints.

Making Ointments

Any herb, fresh or dried, can be used to make an ointment, following this simple recipe: Macerate as much herb as possible in ¾ pint (450ml) of pure olive oil and 2oz (50g) of beeswax for a few hours over a low heat in a bain-marie (double saucepan). After this time the constituents will have been taken up by the oil, and the mixture can be pressed out through a muslin bag and the herb discarded. When the oil is still warm it should be poured into ointment jars, where it will quickly solidify.

Making Creams

Creams can be made up very easily by stirring tinctures, infusions, decoctions or a few drops of essential oil into a base of aqueous cream, which is obtainable from any chemist. Mix two or three drops of *blue camomile* oil into about 2oz (50g) of aqueous cream. Smoothed into the skin, the cream works well on many types of eczema.

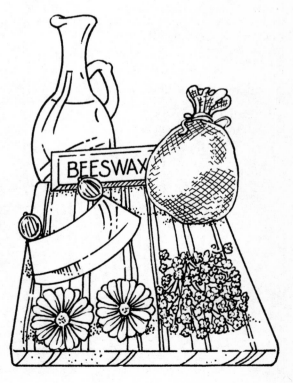

Compresses

Soak a clean cloth or flannel in a hot or cold infusion or decoction, a dilute tincture or water with essential oil. Wring it out and apply it to the affected part. It can work marvels for a bad headache, abdominal colic, period pain, backache, swollen or aching joints, or varicose veins. The treatment needs to be repeated several times for good effect.

Poultices

These are similar to compresses but involve using the herb itself rather than an extract of it.

Making a Poultice

Place the herb, fresh or dried, between two pieces of gauze. If you use fresh leaves, stems and roots, they need to be bruised before being applied. If the herbs are dry, add a little hot water to make either powdered or finely chopped herbs into a paste. Use a light cotton bandage to bind the gauze poultice to the affected part and keep it warm with a hot-water bottle. *Cabbage* leaves used in this way can work wonders for painful arthritic joints, and a bran poultice can swiftly relieve mastitis.

Linaments

A rubbing oil or linament consists of extracts of herbs in an oil or alcohol base, or a mixture of herbal oils and alcohol tinctures of the required herbs. They are used in massage to relax or stimulate muscles and ligaments or to soothe away pain from inflammation or injury. They are intended to be absorbed by the skin to reach the affected part, and so they often contain stimulating essential oils or *cayenne* to increase local circulation.

Oils

Essential oils can be readily obtained from many different sources, including health food shops, and mail-order companies. They are pure oils extracted from aromatic plants by a process of steam distillation, and for this reason it is highly impracticable if not impossible to prepare them at home.

Making Herbal Oils

It is possible to make herbal oils by infusing finely chopped herbs in pure vegetable oil (use olive, sunflower seed or almond oil) for about two weeks. The herbs and oil should be placed in a glass jar with a tight-fitting lid, placed on a sunny window-sill and shaken twice daily. The oil will gradually take up the constituents of the plant, as you will observe by macerating *St John's wort* in oil: the oil will gradually turn a deep red, when it is known as 'heart of Jesus oil'. The oil is healing for cuts and sores and, when massaged in, for painful nerve conditions such as trigeminal neuralgia and shingles. After a minimum of two weeks the oil can be filtered off and the remainder of the herb squeezed through a muslin bag to extract the last drops of oil. It should be stored in an airtight, dark bottle to retain its therapeutic value for a maximum length of time.

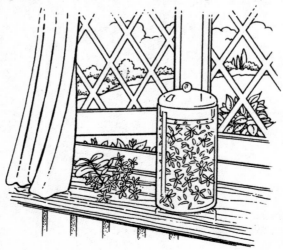

CHAPTER 4

STARTING YOUR OWN HERB GARDEN

Perhaps the most pleasing of all ways to enjoy the benefits of herbs is simply being in their midst, either by growing them in the garden or walking among them in the countryside. On a warm spring or summer day you can inhale the fragrance of *lavender*, *roses*, *thyme*, *rosemary* and *sage* in the garden, or of *elderflowers* or *blackthorn* flowers as you pass down a country lane. The sheer enjoyment of their beauty, as you breathe in their delicate fragrances, brings healing to different aspects of your being that goes far beyond the realms of pharmacological constituents.

Growing your own herbs can bring a great deal of pleasure, and the fresh herbs will provide an instant medicine chest from spring to autumn, while other herbs gathered during this time can be dried or frozen to provide remedies through the winter months.

When you are planning where to site your herb garden, bear in mind that most herbs like sunny positions, ideally facing south and sheltered to the north and east from the cold, particularly from the frost and wind. The closer your herb garden is to the kitchen door, the more likely you will be to use the herbs that you have so carefully nurtured.

If at all possible, the ground in your herb garden should slope down slightly towards the south, so that those herbs that require a sunnier position can be planted at the top and those that prefer less sun and damper soil can go at the bottom. If you decide to plant your herbs either among your flower borders or in your vegetable garden, make sure that they are not shaded from the sun by taller plants.

Most herbs will grow well in almost any soil and any garden, but they generally thrive in a light, well-drained soil. Some herbs – *marjoram*, *oregano* and *thyme*, for instance – love chalky soil, while others – such as *mint*, *camomile*, *angelica* and *lemon balm* – grow better on heavier soils.

There are lots of different forms your herb garden can take, and you can use as much or as little space as you wish. If you live in a town, or if your garden is small, herbs can be grown successfully on a patio, among paving slabs, in tubs, pots (including strawberry pots), urns, old sinks, in hanging baskets or in humble window boxes, as long as they are watered frequently during dry spells.

If you have enough space, time and energy, it can be fun to follow a traditional pattern of the kind that was used in the past in monastery or physic gardens. The best-known design for a formal herb garden, which was popular during Elizabethan times, is the knot garden. Choose low-growing herbs, with contrasting leaf colours, textures and flower shapes, and plant them in rows that interlace with each other to give the appearance of a knotted rope.

A semi-formal herb bed is an easy way to keep a herb garden looking neat and tidy. Paths made from brick, paving stones, gravel or concrete slabs can be used between the beds to make the herbs easily accessible and the garden very attractive. It is wise in any such garden to restrict the growth of invasive roots such as those of *tarragon* or *mint* by putting pieces of slate or tile on end in the ground around the plant.

Herbs planted between vegetables or flowers are not only very attractive but are also beneficial. A row of *mint* between young cabbages will help keep down whitefly; *summer savory* among broad beans will help prevent blackfly; strawberries benefit from nearby *borage* and *sage*; *mint*, *thyme* and *rosemary* are good for brassicas; and *marigold* and *garlic* will help prevent disease and infestation by greenfly of any plant, but especially roses. Bees will be encouraged into your garden by *lemon balm* and *parsley*, and *parsley* will also deter greenfly.

SOWING AND PROPAGATION OF HERBS

Some herbs – *basil*, *coriander*, *marigold*, *dill*, *borage*, *anise* and *parsley*, for example – can be treated as annuals, and seeds should be sown each spring, usually around the end of April or in early May. Plant the seeds close together in

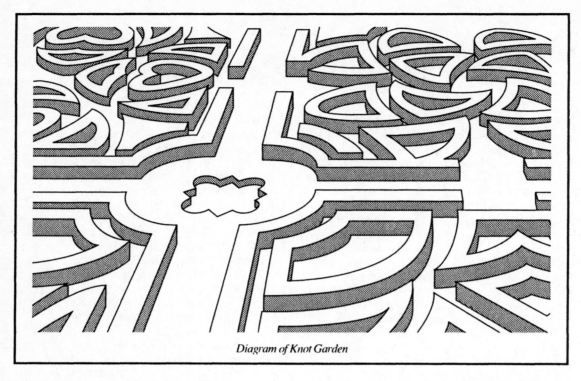

Diagram of Knot Garden

the bed, thin out the seedlings, but leave the plants close enough so that they can support each other as they grow.

In the past, and increasingly today, the phases of the moon have been taken into consideration when sowing seeds and transplanting seedlings. These activities should always be done when the moon is waxing, never when it is waning.

Herbs that are not annuals can be easily propagated by cuttings taken during the summer. *Rosemary, lavender, sage, thyme, hyssop* and *wormwood* fall into this category. Take a cutting 3–4in (7.5–10cm) long from the previous year's growth, trim it just beneath a node (the point at which leaves grow from a stem), dip it in hormone rooting powder if you wish and put it into a pot of potting compost or equal parts of sand and a growing medium. Spray your cuttings with water in the evenings until the roots have formed. Once the cuttings have rooted, you can plant them out where you want them in your herb garden or pot them on for transplanting in the following spring. Hardwood cuttings can be put straight into open ground in the summer as long as they are watered well and frequently until the roots are established and they are protected from too much sun and

wind. You can also take cuttings in late autumn and keep them over winter in a greenhouse or cold frame, ready for planting out in the spring.

Some herbs can be propagated by root division – *mint, lemon balm, chives, tarragon* and *marjoram* can be divided and replanted in either spring or autumn.

HARVESTING HERBS FROM YOUR GARDEN

First establish which part of the plant you need for your medicine. Leaves and flowers should be gathered just as the plant is bursting into bloom, on a dry day once the dew has dried. A flat basket is the best container to collect herbs in as it makes it easier to avoid bruising or crushing the leaves or flowers.

During the growing season leaves and flowers should be gathered and used fresh, ideally straight from the garden. Harvest some extra ones for drying or freezing to last you through the winter months – particularly those that might be useful for winter colds and coughs, such as *thyme, oregano, ground ivy, coltsfoot* and *hyssop*, and for children's fevers, such as *yarrow, mint* and *elderflowers*.

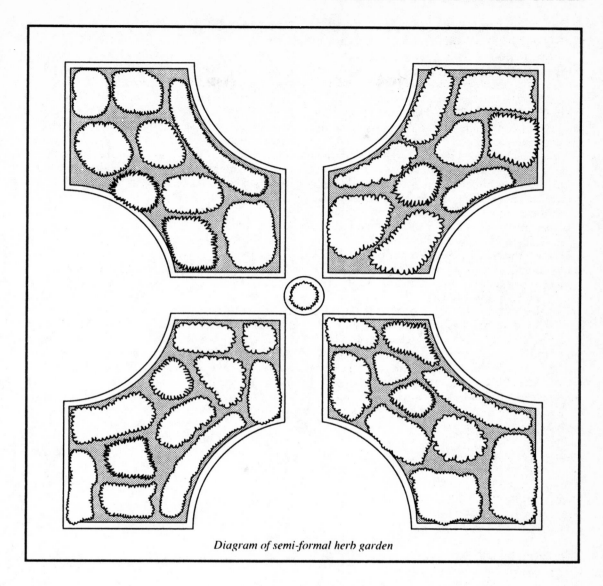

Diagram of semi-formal herb garden

Seeds are collected once they have formed, and it is best to cut off the whole flowerhead when harvesting them, tie it up in a paper bag and hang it upside-down in a dry, well-ventilated place. The seeds will drop into the bag as the flowerhead dries.

Roots and rhizomes (the root-like stems of some species) are normally collected in autumn or spring, once the aerial parts of the plant have died down or before they shoot up and while the plants' energies are under the ground.

In general, when harvesting, choose plants that look as healthy and vibrant as possible. Select those that are free from disease and infestation and those that are growing as far away as possible from busy roads or sprayed fields.

DRYING HERBS

The aim of the drying process is to reduce the moisture in the plant before it starts to die so that it can be stored for a few months without deteriorating and while retaining its therapeutic properties.

The best places for drying herbs are shaded, well-ventilated rooms that are free from

31

moisture or condensation – avoid the kitchen, bathroom, utility room, damp sheds or garages for this reason – and that are at a steady temperature of about 90°F (32°C) – an airing-cupboard is ideal, or you could use a shaded greenhouse as long as the temperature does not fall below 72°F (22°C). If the atmosphere is too cold the plants will reabsorb moisture from the air and take too long to dry.

Dry the herbs as soon as possible after you have harvested them. Spread out the aerial parts – leaves and flowers – so that there is plenty of space between them on a tray and cover them with muslin or fine wire netting, or place them in a shallow box without a lid. Turn them frequently – once or twice on the first day and once daily thereafter. Some herbs may be hung upside-down in small bunches from hooks or beams. Tie the bunches loosely with string so that air can circulate between the stalks. If the bunches are too tightly fastened, the stalks may rot and go mouldy. *Rosemary, sage, wormwood, mint* and *lavender* can all be hung to dry.

Barks, roots and rhizomes should be washed thoroughly, patted dry and chopped up before being spread out to dry.

STORING HERBS

Crumble the leafy herbs between your hands, remove the stalks and twigs and store them in wooden or cardboard boxes (shoe boxes are very useful), jars with airtight lids or paper bags. Roots, rhizomes and barks should be broken up into small pieces and stored in a similar way. Carefully label all herbs before they are dry. If you find moisture inside one of the containers you are using, tip out all the herbs on to clean paper and leave them to dry for a little while longer.

FREEZING HERBS

Herbs, particularly those with soft leaves, such as *marjoram, borage, comfrey, coriander, fennel, basil, lemon balm, mint* and *parsley*, are ideal for freezing. Pick the leaves or flowers, wash them, chop them or leave them whole, and place them to freeze in small plastic bags. Alternatively, place individual flowers or chopped leaves in ice-cube trays and freeze them; you can then pack the cubes in small bags to store in the freezer.

PART II
HERBAL BABY CARE

CHAPTER 5

THE FIRST FEW MONTHS OF LIFE

Caring for your infant or child begins not at the moment of birth but several months even before conception. The future health of your child is closely linked not only to its phase of life as a foetus in your womb but also to the health of the sperm and egg that created it. A healthy ovum, fertilized by a healthy sperm, will provide the best possible genetic inheritance and lay the foundation of the child's basic constitution, which will determine much of its future health and well-being.

Ideally, both parents should be in the best of health when the baby is conceived. Try to plan ahead for your pregnancy and visit your doctor for a general check-up or make an appointment with your local Foresight practitioner (see Appendix 5 for addresses) and give yourselves the opportunity to right any imbalances or illnesses that could pose potential risks to your child.

During the preconceptual period and throughout pregnancy, herbal remedies can provide valuable medicine to be used both therapeutically and preventatively. Herbs can be taken with great benefit to enhance general health and well-being, as well as to right specific imbalances you may be aware of. Herbs are of particular value during pregnancy, and they have been used since time began by women all over the world to ensure optimum health and to prepare for the birth, as well as to help them through various difficulties that may arise, such as nausea, heartburn, backache, urinary problems, long childbirth or post-natal problems.

As the move towards 'natural' pregnancy and childbirth and away from medical intervention develops, an increasing number of women are looking towards the time-proved safety of natural remedies to enhance their general well-being and treat specific imbalances or disorders they may have without risk of side-effects to either themselves or to their unborn offspring. Herbal remedies are gaining in respect and popularity among many such women. Nutrition and plant remedies can be used therapeutically and preventatively, and, with the exception of a few notable herbs, they are perfectly safe to use throughout pregnancy, childbirth and post-natally during breast-feeding. When used with knowledge and understanding herbs can be taken to help ensure a straightforward delivery, free from stress and medical intervention.

Several herbs can be used during pregnancy, in childbirth and post-natally. Herbs such as *raspberry leaves*, *false unicorn root*, *motherwort*, *blue cohosh* and *squaw vine* can be taken in preparation for the birth to help ease delivery. Others such as *black haw*, *cramp bark* and *wild yam* can be used during childbirth to speed and ease delivery, either to strengthen ineffectual contractions or to relax tense, over-painful contractions, both of which can delay the birth and thereby lead to possible complications. There are herbs for nausea, urinary problems, nervous tension, bowel problems, varicose veins, anaemia, exhaustion, post-natal depression, to enhance breast-feeding, and to remedy any breast discomfort and inflammation during feeding. Herbs can also be used post-natally to restore both mother – and father, if necessary – and baby after the birth. They can help speed recovery of energy and repair of tissues damaged by bruising or tearing during delivery. There are several famous tonics for women after childbirth, notably *Chinese angelica*, *false unicorn root* or *raspberry leaves* taken with *ginger*, *cloves* or *cinnamon*, which can be used for general post-natal care, restoration of energy and to help ease the transition into parenthood. Others can be given to the baby, perhaps used in massage or bath water, to help the new-born infant adjust to life outside the womb.

BREAST-FEEDING

Being born involves an enormous transition from one state of dependency inside the womb, to another outside the womb, where the baby needs to be fed, nurtured, kept warm, secure and loved. Breast-feeding provides a wonderful means of providing nurture on all levels to ease the transition from one world to another. To many it is a vital part of mothering. In fact, much research has proved the beneficial effects of breast-feeding on the baby's emotional as well as physical development, especially the breast-feeding and skin contact that occurs immediately after the birth. Some researchers in Uganda found that babies born in hospitals continued to produce birth-stress hormones in considerable quantity for between eight and twelve weeks after the birth, compared with one or two days in naturally delivered babies. The same difference in hormone production was also found in American and European children between those born naturally and those delivered in hospitals. The reason was that the separation from the mother at birth that occurs in hospitals meant that none of the signals of birth completion happen, and the baby's adrenal glands maintain the state of alert that occurs during the birth. This continued state of alert can cause exhaustion and prolonged sleeping or crying.[1]

The Advantages of Breast-feeding

It is worth considering the advantages of breast-feeding as opposed to bottle-feeding – and there are many.

• Breast milk helps to protect the baby against infections, certain diseases and developmental problems.

• Particularly important is colostrum, which contains antibodies to many of the diseases the mother has had or has been immunized against and which provides the baby with many of the substances needed for the normal maturation of the baby's own immune system, including gammalinoleic acid (see page 69). It also contains substances that help to protect against gastro-enteritis and diarrhoea. In fact, if you breast-feed for at least thirteen weeks, you will help to protect your child from gastro-enteritis for the first two years of life.

• Lactose, the sugar present in breast milk, supports the growth of beneficial bacteria in the baby's gut, at the expense of pathogenic ones, and so helps to prevent the development of infection. Commercial baby milks contain glucose, maltose or dextrose, which are easier for pathogenic bacteria to use and which encourage a sweet tooth as they are much sweeter than lactose.

• Breast milk also helps to protect against chest and urinary infections. Infective diarrhoea, chest infections, meningitis and septicaemia are more common in bottle-fed babies all over the world, and in some undeveloped countries infant mortality is far higher among bottle-fed than among breast-fed babies – bottle-fed babies in the Philippines, for example, are forty times more likely to die than breast-fed ones.[2]

• Breast milk contains certain sugars, called oligosaccharides, which are carried from the baby's gut to the lining of the lungs, where they prevent pathogenic organisms, such as haemophilus bacteria, from causing pneumonia and bronchiolitus from damaging the lungs.

• Allergies tend to occur less in breast-fed babies, especially if there is a family history of allergy, when it is best to breast-feed exclusively for as long as you can. Breast milk helps to boost the baby's immunity. A baby's immune system is immature for the first four to six months, and during this time any foods that are given can affect the development of allergies later in life, even in adulthood. Symptoms of allergy in a baby may include colic, constipation, diarrhoea, crying, nappy rash, dry skin and dermatitis, catarrh and convulsions.

• Disorders such as coeliac disease (see page 141) (and probably ulcerative colitis and

Crohn's disease), are less likely to occur in breast-fed babies. Bottle-fed babies who develop infective diarrhoea may have further bowel problems caused by inflammation of the lining of the gut, which can leave residual damage. This can lead to poor absorption of nutrients, particularly sugars, and to sugar intolerance. Unabsorbed sugars remain in the gut, further irritating it and attracting water, causing more diarrhoea. The sugary environment in the gut attracts bacteria, and a vicious circle results, weakening the baby and causing lowered resistance to further disease, and threatening dehydration if diarrhoea continues, especially in a hot climate.

• Nutritionally, breast milk is the perfect food for babies. It is as obviously designed to suit a baby's needs as cow's milk is for calves. In fact, cow's milk has to be modified considerably to make it suitable for feeding babies, but the constituents can never be identical to breast milk. Certain enzymes and hormones in breast milk do not correspond with those in cow's milk, which either can only be used by calves or are destroyed in processing. The nutritional composition of breast milk is ideal for building the body of a human infant, especially during the first few weeks when it doubles its birth weight and develops its first co-ordinated movements.

• The physical relationship between a breast-feeding mother and her baby is quite miraculous – by sucking a baby calls for nutritional supplies, and breast milk is produced as a response. The more the child demands and sucks, the more milk is supplied and the baby gets all that is needed. This is hard to gauge if you are bottle-feeding.

• During the first five days after the birth, the mother secretes colostrum, for the next five days the milk changes into transitional milk and after that mature milk is supplied. The character of the milk also changes during the course of a feed in the same breast, and milk is not necessarily the same in both breasts. During the first 5 minutes of an average feed of about 15 minutes, a baby will take around 60 per cent of the total milk in the breast, 60 per cent of the protein and carbohydrate, over 40 per cent of the fat and more than half the total energy. During the next 6 minutes, the ratio of

fat to other nutrients increases considerably, and the baby feels more satisfied.

• The ratio of fat to protein and carbohydrate in breast milk is particularly suited to humans, whose brains develop far more quickly than in animals. Different ratios of nutrients are needed to build the brain and nervous system than are required to build other body tissues. For example, more essential fatty acids are needed for the brain and nervous system and more protein is needed for body tissues. Cow's milk contains three or four times as much protein as human milk, and this corresponds to the difference in the bulk of a cow's body compared with a human body, even in those who are fat. In contrast, breast milk contains the least protein of all animal milks investigated, but it contains ten times as much essential fatty acids, necessary for building the brain and nervous system. It is interesting that a rhinoceros weighs a ton at the age of four while a human child weighs about 44lb (20kg) at the same age. By the age of four, the human brain weighs $3\frac{1}{2}$lb (1.5kg) and is already formed, and a rhino's brain weighs about $10\frac{1}{2}$oz (300g) and you can fit it into the palm of your hand.[3]

• Breast milk is more easily digested and assimilated than formulae based on cow's milk, so that breast-fed babies tend to have fewer digestive upsets and disorders such as colic and constipation. Not only this, but the absorption of the other vital nutrients is also influenced by the kind of milk a baby has. The predominance of lactose in breast milk means that when it is broken down by bacteria it becomes lactic acid. Vitamin C and several B vitamins are easily destroyed in the body unless they are held in acid until they reach the bloodstream. Iron, phosphorus, calcium and other essential minerals can only dissolve in acid. Therefore, because of the greater proportion of lactic acid produced in the intestines of breast-fed babies, they absorb far more vitamin C, vitamin B, iron, calcium and so on than bottle-fed ones, even if the formula contains the same amount of nutrients to start with.

• Bottle-fed babies tend to put on more body weight than breast-fed ones, and this may predispose them to colds and chest problems, as well as to being overweight later on in life. They may also be more prone to the development of heart and arterial disease and diabetes.

● Emotionally and developmentally, breast-feeding also has its advantages. Breast-feeding means that a baby will be held close to mother for some time during the day and night, especially if you demand-feed. Bottle-fed babies tend to be fed every three or four hours, and to sleep more, often away from their mothers in cots. With the holding that accompanies breast-feeding comes bonding, and nurture that far exceeds the nutritional value of the milk.

● Research has indicated that, perhaps because of this nurture and bonding, coupled with the nutritional components that favour brain development, breast-fed children walk sooner, are more intelligent and do better at school, and are less likely to be jealous, insecure and aggressive, than those who are bottle-fed. A baby who can determine its own supply of nutrients simply by sucking, especially whenever it needs to in unrestricted feeding, may feel more powerful and secure than one who is fed a pre-determined amount at regular intervals through the day.

● Research has also shown that the early ability of the new-born baby to use its eyes is affected by bonding.[4] If there is close eye contact with the mother immediately after the birth, the child develops the ability to use its eyes. If the child is taken away from its mother at birth, it may take several more weeks to establish the ability to use its eyes. If the baby is held by its mother after the birth and there is eye contact, this can be critical in the development of the child's vision – the 45-minute period of alertness after the birth being a most important time when a baby can recognize his or her mother's face if it is about a foot (30cm) away, and then afterwards the baby will recognize her face each time it comes near, and the vision and the bonding process will develop securely hand in hand.

● For a mother too, breast-feeding can give a wonderful feeling of joy and fulfilment, coupled with the pleasure of knowing that her baby is having the best possible nourishment. The close relationship breast-feeding engenders may last for the rest of your lives, and certainly it has been found that breast-feeding mothers are generally less aggressive or hostile, and are less likely to want to control or reject the child.[5]

● Breast-feeding is also much more convenient. The milk is readily available, it requires no preparation, it comes at the right temperature, and it is germ free and full of antibodies to protect the baby against illness and infection. It helps the mother's uterus to contract back to its normal size, and it uses up excess fat. There is also evidence to show that prolonged breast-feeding can also reduce the incidence of breast cancer.

Most women are eager to breast-feed their babies, but it is not always as straightforward as you would think – there is quite an art to breast-feeding that in the past midwives would have been able to teach. Many women start and continue until they develop such sore nipples that they cannot go on; others stop through lack of sufficient milk. But there is help – preventative and therapeutic – for most breast-feeding problems, as well as more practical advice available in books and from midwives and health visitors, so don't give up too easily!

The sooner after the birth you start to breast-feed, the easier it will be in the long term. So keep your baby with you, lie him on your abdomen and let him find the breast, or put him gently to the breast, and you will find that he will be much less stressed than if he is taken away to be washed and weighed. Less stress will mean easier breast-feeding and will start your relationship off on the right foot. If you have had pain killers during the birth you may find the baby very sleepy, and you may find it takes a while for him to suck strongly. Don't worry, it will happen in time.

Let your baby determine how long and how often you will feed – this will make for a plentiful supply of milk and prevent engorgement of the breasts, which can be extremely uncomfortable. Drink plenty of fluids to keep up your milk supply, and rest as much as you can so that your energy does not become drained. Your diet needs to be as nutritious as it was during pregnancy, to supply both your own and your baby's needs and to maintain your energy and aid recovery after the birth. Your body will provide the breast milk preferentially with nutrients, and so any dietary deficiencies will affect you before it will diminish the quality of the milk.

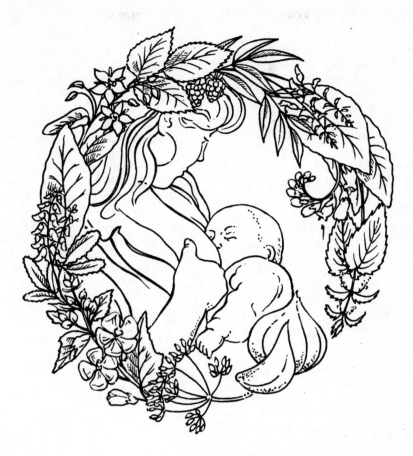

Poor Milk Supply

Some women find it hard to get milk production established; others find that they cannot maintain a plentiful supply to satisfy a hungry baby. There are several possible reasons for this. A poor diet or a reduction in your intake of food if you are trying to lose weight after the birth may mean that you get tired and run-down, and this will affect your milk supply. Exhaustion after a long birth may prevent breast-feeding from being well established in the first week or two, and overtiredness from broken nights or trying to do too much may cause milk supply to dwindle once it does get going. The anxiety and tension associated with feeding are very common problems, and they inhibit the let-down reflex and so stop the flow of milk. Many mothers worry about being able to produce enough milk to satisfy and nourish the baby, often even before the baby is born.

Since breast milk is supplied on a supply and demand basis, if you feel your production is scanty, try drinking more fluids and feeding the baby more frequently. Let your baby decide how long and how often to feed, not you. The hormone prolactin is responsible for producing milk. When the baby sucks at the breast, the stimulus is given to produce more prolactin and so more milk is made. Once the baby starts to suckle, the hormone oxytocin is released into the bloodstream, and when it reaches the breasts it causes the tiny muscles around each milk-producing cell to contract and squeeze the milk down a system of ducts which lead to the nipple. This is known as the let-down reflex, and this can be inhibited if you feel tense, shy or embarrassed about breast-feeding. If you have problems with the let-down reflex, it is probably best to feed your baby quietly, on your own, so that you can concentrate wholly on the baby and relax properly. Put on your favourite music, have a warm relaxing drink or an aromatic bath – you can always take the baby with you and feed in the bath.

Herbs to Increase and Enhance the Milk Supply

Many herbs have been used successfully for centuries to stimulate milk production and to enhance and enrich the milk supply once started: *aniseed, borage, caraway seeds, centaury, cinnamon, comfrey, dill, false unicorn root, fennel seeds, fenugreek, goat's rue, holy thistle, garlic, marshmallow, melilot, milk thistle, milkwort, nettles, raspberry leaves, saw palmetto, vervain* and *vitex (chaste tree)*.

These can be taken as tinctures, but are best taken as teas, frequently through the day to ensure that you keep up your fluid intake.

Any of these herbs can be combined together to suit your taste, and you can alter the prescription when you feel the need for a change. I have always found an infusion of equal parts of *borage, raspberry leaves, nettles, holy thistle* and *cinnamon* to be delicious and very effective.

An infusion of equal parts of *fennel seeds, goat's rue, marshmallow, vervain, fenugreek* and *vitex* makes a more spicy-tasting tea, but one that is equally effective. Make sure you crush the seeds well before infusing them in boiling water.

You could also try spicy *raspberry leaf* tea with honey and ½ teaspoon (2–3ml) of a mixture of powdered *ginger, cinnamon* and *cloves*. Start to take this as soon as the baby is born – it is very reviving when you feel tired or are recovering from the birth, and it tastes delicious.

Many of these herbs are very nutritious – *nettles, marshmallow, comfrey, raspberry leaves, borage* and *garlic*, for example – while some, such as *vervain, borage, holy thistle* and *raspberry leaves* have relaxant properties, which help allay any anxiety while breast-feeding. Others such as *fennel, caraway, cinnamon, aniseed* and *dill*, are warming and antispasmodic, helping to relieve muscle tension. *Borage* is to me a particularly special herb. It has beautiful little blue flowers, which you can add to fruit juices and salads and use to decorate puddings. The flowers contain calcium and phosphorus, and they were used traditionally to 'gladden the heart' and lift depression. They are particularly useful if you feel sad or regretful when it is time to wean your baby.

Vitex seeds work on the pituitary gland to stimulate secretion of the hormone prolactin, which governs production of breast milk. *Saw palmetto* berries promote the proper functioning of the mammary glands in the breast. Take three or five berries daily in the last month of pregnancy and while nursing.

Not only will these nutritious and balancing herbs benefit you, the feeding mother, but they will pass through the milk to your baby. Many of the herbs that enhance milk supply have a high volatile oil content, which is antiseptic and antibiotic as well as antispasmodic. These will not only boost the baby's immune system but also help digestion and reduce any tendency to tension or colic. In addition *thyme, ground ivy, rosemary, camomile, peppermint, yarrow, marjoram, elderflowers* and *garlic* can all be used specifically for minor infections such as coughs or colds or for digestive problems (see pages 72 and 129). These can be taken as teas or added regularly to cooking or salads.

Essential Oils Essential oils can also be used to enhance milk supply. Choose either *fennel, geranium* or *clary sage* and use about 10 drops in 1fl oz (30ml) of almond oil and massage it into each breast with circular movements once a day.

Diet to Enhance Milk Supply

It is important to eat well to maintain your milk supply, now you really are eating for two – in fact you need about 500 extra calories a day. You can also enhance and enrich your milk supply by the foods that you eat every day. Maize, oats, barley, peas and beans and pulses will produce plentiful and nutritious milk. Onions and leeks enrich the milk and have antiseptic qualities. Nuts, especially walnuts and almonds, and seeds, such as sunflower, sesame, linseed, celery and fenugreek seeds, can be sprinkled on stews and salads or roasted and eaten as a tasty snack to stimulate milk production. Most raw fruits, especially bananas, blackcurrants, rosehips, grapes, pears, peaches and apples, and most raw vegetables, particularly carrots, watercress, chicory, as well as *dandelion* and *comfrey* leaves, and green herbs such as *coriander, borage, land cress, alfalfa* and *spring onions* are also beneficial.

Remedies for Sore, Cracked Nipples

It is very common for your nipples to become very sensitive during the first week after the baby is born, but after that the tenderness generally subsides, although in some women it can persist for a few weeks, especially when the baby starts feeding. However, do not give up too easily – there are practical guidelines to prevent sore nipples, and to help them once they start to feel tender or bruised, or start to crack.

Are You Feeding Properly? Sore nipples are often caused because the baby is not latched on to the breast properly, so it is important to make sure your baby gets on to the breast correctly right from the start. First, make sure that you feel comfortable; use pillows to sit on if your perineum feels sore or to place on your lap to raise the baby to the breast. Rest your feet on a stool if you need to. Consciously relax and let go of any tension you feel in your body. Breathe slowly and relaxedly. Hold the baby so that the head is tilted back and the chin is resting against your breast, and then, when the baby sucks, he will be able to get the areola of the breast into the mouth properly. You will know that he is latched on properly when you see the ears moving as he or she feeds. If the cheeks go in and out, the baby is not on properly. When feeding properly, he will feed in spurts and then rest. When the baby has had enough, he will stop feeding and may continue just to comfort suck. If he or she starts chewing the nipple and the cheeks go in and out, take the baby off the breast, as this could make your nipples very sore. You could give a dummy if the baby cries and wants to suck but only comfort sucks when offered the breast.

Let the Baby Feed Unrestrictedly. This is most important in the first few days when the colostrum comes through, because it starts the baby's digestive system working and contains all the protein, fats, vitamins and minerals the baby needs. If the baby is able to feed sufficiently, he or she will feel satisfied and sleep for long hours in between feeds. This will give your nipples a rest and a chance to heal. If the baby is taken off the breast, not quite satisfied, he or she will soon wake again for another feed, and if this happens a few times, will suck harder on the nipple to make sure he or she gets all he needs quickly before being taken off the breast again. This could make the nipple sore.

Don't Wash Your Breasts Too Frequently. Especially do not wash with soap, as you will wash the natural oils out of the nipple and make the skin more prone to damage. Once a day is quite enough. Let the nipples dry naturally after each feed: you can express a little milk and rub it in and allow it to dry on the nipple to help protect the skin. Keep your nipples dry between feeds by using breast pads: so that your skin does not become soggy, change the pads when they get damp. Start each feed on a different side from the last one, and change your position frequently so that the pressure on the areola is not all in the same place.

Expose Your Nipples to the Air. Do this as often as possible, especially after feeds. Try to avoid wearing a bra and breast pads at night, even though you may get quite wet, to allow the air to circulate around the breasts.

Ointment for Sore Nipples

There are several remedies that you can apply to the nipples to help prevent them from becoming sore. Buttermilk, honey and *comfrey ointment* will help to keep the skin on the nipple supple. Massage the nipple with these before the birth to get it used to being touched frequently. Alternatively, you could use *calendula* or *chickweed* ointment, *thick honey*, *almond oil*, *wheatgerm oil* or *rose water*, as preventative measures, and to heal the nipple once it has become sore or cracked. One drop of *rose oil* in 2 teaspoons of almond oil is also very effective and smells beautiful. *Comfrey ointment* is the best tissue healer there is. You can also use fresh *mullein leaves*, boiled slowly in milk for 10 minutes and cooled. Wrap them in a piece of gauze and apply for 10–20 minutes, or use *mullein ointment*. All these remedies can be applied frequently, after feeding.

If your nipples become so sore that you find feeding difficult, make sure you express any excess milk, to avoid the breasts becoming engorged.

Remedies for Engorgement of the Breast

Some engorgement tends to occur between two and five days after the birth, when the milk starts to come in, but, luckily, it is usually temporary. It is related to the increased blood supply to the breasts and excess fluid due to the increased activity in the breasts. When breasts become engorged they can feel very hot, swollen, hard and painful, and they tend to flatten the nipple, making it hard for the baby to suckle. This obviously can cause further engorgement and discomfort for the poor mother, and make for a very hungry, unhappy and tired baby.

General Self-Help Try to ease the extra fluid in the breast away from the nipple with your fingertips, so that the nipple stands out for the baby to latch on to. If you let the baby feed on demand from the beginning, you will probably find that the engorgement that occurs in the first few days is mild and passes easily. If the problem is persistent, you can try applying ice-cold flannels after feeding to constrict the blood vessels and help the swelling to subside. Washing your breasts with warm water just before feeding will help to get the milk flow going, as will vigorous arm-swinging exercises. The breasts will feel better as soon as the milk is flowing properly as your baby feeds, and the breasts are emptied.

Infusions and Decoctions To help reduce swelling and excess fluid (oedema) in the breast take teas three times daily made from *blackcurrant leaves*, *cleavers* or *marigold*. A decoction of *dandelion root* is also helpful. A hot compress of decoction of *poke root* or infusion of *cleavers*, can be applied frequently to the breasts, or if it is the right time of year, you can place fresh *rhubarb* or *cabbage leaves* inside the bra for about three hours – these work wonderfully well and can reduce congestion and return the breast to a normal size within a very short time.

Essential Oils Essential oils of *fennel, rose, lavender* and *geranium* can be used with good effect. Add a few drops of oil to a bowl of hot water, and apply hot compresses frequently to the breast to ease swelling and discomfort. You can also use a few drops of *rose* or *peppermint* oil in *mullein* tincture and mixed into aqueous cream to rub into the breast.

Compress A pleasant remedy for engorged breasts can be prepared using 5 tablespoons of *basil* and 1¾ pints (1 litre) of *rose water*. Leave the basil to macerate in the rose water for 48 hours, shaking from time to time. Apply warm compresses soaked in the liquid frequently to the breast.

Remedies for Inflamed Breasts and Mastitis

It is important to treat (or hopefully prevent) sore nipples as soon as they become sensitive so that the breasts do not become engorged for any length of time. It is also vital to reduce any engorgement that develops as quickly as you can so that the breast does not become inflamed through a blocked duct, which will cause even more pain and swelling. If you have flushing or redness of the skin on the breast you may well have a blocked duct. If this is not treated an infection may set in, known as mastitis, which can cause a sharp rise in temperature, influenza-like symptoms, tenderness, usually on the outer part of the breast, and flushing of the skin. Feed as often as you can to help reduce the engorgement, and express any milk left in the breast after each feed.

Remedies for Mastitis with Fever

If you have a fever, drink plenty of fluid; teas of *yarrow* and *elderflower* mixed with *cleavers* are best. *Dandelion root* tea is an effective remedy for hot, red inflamed breasts and mastitis and is specific in China for mastitis. You could also take equal parts of *golden seal, ginger* and *black cohosh* as tea or tincture three or four times a day. *Poke root, cleavers, marigold, mullein* and *dandelion root* can be used as strong teas or dilute tinctures to reduce congestion and inflammation.

External Treatment For external use you could pound up *lady's mantle* and *sweet violet leaves* with a little hot water, add some honey and spread this on a piece of gauze and apply it as a poultice to the breasts. Cling film is useful for holding it in place and keeping it warm. Alternatively, you could make a poultice from warm cooked *bran, linseed* or *slippery elm*. Mixing these with a little *lobelia tincture* makes them more effective. You could also use *linseed oil* with a little *spirit of camphor* or a few drops of *geranium oil* to rub into the breast. Distilled *witch hazel*, buttermilk, *St John's wort, poke root, comfrey* and *raspberry leaves* are all useful.

● Hand and foot baths can also be effective: a *camomile* or *eucalyptus* foot bath every two hours will help bring down fever, while *lavender* will help resolve the infection.

Herbs for Reducing Milk Flow and Weaning

When you decide (or your baby decides for you) to stop breast-feeding, it is best to wean gradually to cause the least discomfort to yourself through engorged breasts and flooding, for once you stop feeding it can take quite a while for the milk glands to stop working. If you take it slowly, you should have no problems weaning, but there are remedies to help reduce milk flow if your circumstances force you to stop feeding more abruptly. These should never, of course, be taken when you are breast-feeding. *Red sage*, *herb Robert* and *periwinkle* all help to control over-abundant milk and to dry up milk when weaning. Cut down on your fluid consumption and eat plenty of *garden mint*, *sorrel* and *sage* with your meals. A glass of carrot juice first thing in the morning has also been said to reduce breast milk.

Hazardous Substances and Breast Milk

Drugs Women who are breast-feeding need to be particularly careful about taking drugs, most of which will pass through into the breast milk and to the baby. What may be a standard dose of a drug to you, is likely to be a massive dose to your small baby. The effects of some drugs on the baby have been investigated, others have not – but before you take any, it is best to check their possible effect on the baby.[7]

Dietary Factors Other harmful substances may be taken in through your daily diet and passed into your breast milk – your tap water may contain toxins such as pesticides; your fruit and vegetables may contain herbicides and insecticides; your fish, eggs and meat may contain even higher levels of these – so vegetarian mothers fare best and have been found to have lower levels of insecticides in their breast milk than meat and fish eaters.

Caffeine and Alcohol Other substances that can affect breast milk include caffeine, which occurs in tea, coffee, cocoa, chocolate and cola drinks and which may make your baby restless and agitated and cause difficulty sleeping; and alcohol, which can cause colic, irritability and restlessness in a baby. Alcohol can also affect the let-down reflex by inhibiting the production of oxytocin, which blocks the reflex and thus causes an inability to feed.

Nicotine Nicotine from cigarettes can also interfere with the let-down reflex, and it can accumulate in breast milk, possibly causing nausea or vomiting, restlessness and circulatory problems in babies of heavy smokers. Of course, passive smoking is worth taking into consideration, too. Smoking can increase the effects of caffeine.

Environmental Toxins Toxins such as pesticides, dioxin, PCBs and furans from the atmosphere can be inhaled, passed into a mother's bloodstream and then into her milk. You should, therefore, avoid crops that have been sprayed recently and try not to inhale vapours from paints, adhesives, protective wood coatings, dry-cleaning solvents and so on. Vegetarians and vegans have been found to absorb fewer toxins than meat eaters, because toxins tend to accumulate in animal flesh. So it is best to avoid or to eat less red meat, dairy produce and animal fats. Pollution from car exhausts and heavy metals such as mercury, aluminium and lead can all pass into the breast milk.

Minimizing contaminants in breast milk

• Eat a vegetarian diet – research has shown that the breast milk of vegetarian mothers contains as much as a half to two-thirds less pesticide residues than milk of average meat-eating women,[7] and that meat is one of the most concentrated sources of contaminants.

• Eat as many organic foods as possible, and scrub other fruit and vegetables well (with biodegradable soap) before eating them.

• Avoid tap water as far as you can and use bottled mineral water.

• Avoid animal fats – use low-fat dairy produce, including cottage cheese, skimmed milk and low-fat yoghurt and make sure you have plenty of essential fatty acids from unrefined vegetable oils, nuts and seeds in your diet.

• Take supplements of brewer's yeast and a multi-mineral and vitamin tablet to help protect your body from contamination and to flush pollutants from the system.

• Use detoxifying herbs to enhance the function of the liver and kidneys in clearing toxins from the system. *Artichoke* leaves, *burdock* root, *celery* seeds, *cleavers*, *dandelion* leaves and root, and *echinacea* are all useful.

43

CHAPTER 6

LOOKING AFTER YOUR BABY

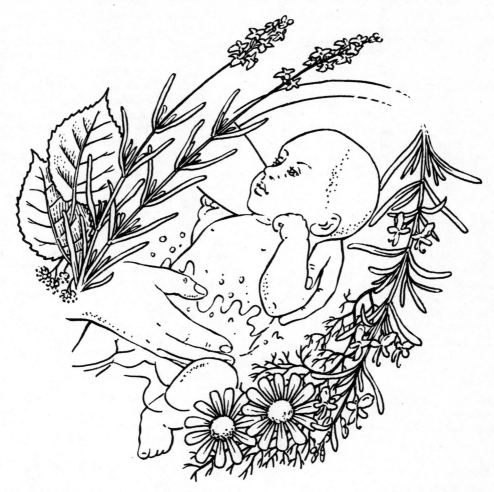

Herbs can be used in all sorts of ways for babies – you can bathe them in herb-scented water, use herbal washes for their eyes, face, and the nappy area to cleanse and protect the skin, massage their feet, tummies and backs with herbal oils, and make weak infusions of herbs for them to drink between feeds (use $\frac{1}{4}$ teaspoon of herb for each cup of boiling water). When you want to administer herbs medicinally to treat a specific problem, you can do so in these ways, or through hand and foot baths, sponging or applying compresses of herbal infusions. In addition, you can use essential oils in vaporizers or in baths, and put a few drops on radia-

tors and light bulbs where the baby is sleeping, so that the baby will inhale them. You can also take herbs yourself, and these will pass through your breast milk to the baby.

BABY BATHS

To bathe your baby, you can use infusions of *rosemary*, *camomile*, *lavender* and *limeflowers*, mixed with tepid water. (Refer to p.26 for further information on how to prepare a herbal bath.) Clean the eyes, face and nappy area with antiseptic infusions of *lavender* or *marigold* so that you do not have to use soap. If the skin looks dirty, especially when the baby starts crawling on hands and knees, you can use coarse oatmeal in a muslin bag, and dilute essential oils or herbal oils of *rosemary, sage, thyme* or *lavender*. Any sore or dry skin can be rubbed with a couple of drops of *lavender oil* in almond oil diluted with *rose water*, so that you do not need to use chemical-based creams.

DRESSING THE UMBILICAL CORD

After the birth, the cord that joins the baby to the placenta is clamped and cut. Over the next ten days it shrinks and drops off. During this time it needs to be cleaned daily as it may get contaminated by urine. You can use antiseptic herbs and oils to dress the umbilical cord. Dilute *oil of cloves* has been widely used in midwifery in the past and can happily be used today. You could also use distilled *witch hazel* or *rosemary tea*. For any redness or inflammation, use *marshmallow tea*, alternated by *tincture of calendula (marigold)*, applied on cotton wool. *Tincture of myrrh* or *echinacea* would also be helpful. These can also be added to the bath water and used to soak gauze to apply between the cord and the nappy.

NAPPY RASH

You can usually avoid nappy rash by washing the baby's bottom with dilute herbal infusions of *lavender, camomile* or *marigold* or with *rose water*. Make sure that baby's skin dries properly – perhaps leave the baby to kick with no nappy on for a while in a warm room or outside in the sunshine. Nappy rash can be caused when damp skin is enclosed for hours, often days or weeks in a wet, chafing nappy without enough air to circulate around it. Before putting a nappy on, rub cream into the nappy area, using herbs in a natural base (see page 27). You could choose from *camomile, chickweed, comfrey* and *marigold*, any of which will be healing and soothing and protect the skin against any corrosive effects of urine and stools.

You can also use herbal oils – *St John's wort oil* is particularly effective. Essential oil of *lavender* or *camomile* in a base of almond oil can also be used. Avoid using talcum power, because this cakes on the skin, holding in the

damp and collecting bacteria, and can make nappy rash worse or introduce a secondary infection.

Causes of Nappy Rash

• When urine and stools in the nappy are left in contact with the skin for too long, the bacteria in the stool break down the urine to release ammonia, which irritates the skin. A red rash round the genitals appears which, if left untreated, can become tight and shiny and may develop pustules. Bacteria breed better in an alkaline environment, which is encouraged by bottle-feeding, than in the more acid stool produced by a breast-fed baby.

• If the rash tends to affect only the skin creases at the top of the thighs, it is probably simply due to not drying the baby adequately after washing or bathing.

• If you use fabric nappies, your baby may develop an allergic reaction to chemicals in the washing powder or fabric conditioner. If this is the cause, the rash will cover most of the area covered by the nappy. Use a non-biological washing powder.

• Monilial infection (thrush) is also a major cause of nappy rash. If the rash begins around

---

Causes of Nappy Rash

☐ Irritation from a wet, chafing nappy on the skin for much of the day
☐ Ammonia released from urine irritating the skin
☐ Not drying the skin properly after washing
☐ Allergic reaction to washing powder, fabric conditioner or rubber in elastic
☐ Atopic eczema
☐ Thrush
☐ Bacterial infection
☐ Herpes
☐ Sensitive skin and a tendency to seborrhoea
☐ Plastic pants, talcum powder and diarrhoea can make the rash worse

---

the anus and spreads over the buttocks and on to the thighs, it could be caused by thrush. Check in the mouth for signs of thrush there too.

● Small blisters on the rash may indicate that nappy rash has weakened the skin's defences and a herpes infection has developed. Any nappy rash can also become secondarily infected with bacteria.

● Nappy rash tends to occur in babies with sensitive skins and those who are prone to seborrhoea, indicated by cradle cap or seborrhoeic dermatitis elsewhere on the skin, very often over the eyebrows and forehead. It may be that nappy rash is the beginning of atopic eczema (see page 144).

● If irritation is caused by urine or stools, diarrhoea tends to make it worse.

● If your baby's skin is red around the waist and top of the legs where elastic or plastic pants have rubbed, it may be that the nappies or pants are too tight or that the skin is sensitive to the rubber in the elastic. Plastic pants also increase the tendency to nappy rash as they hold moisture in the nappy.

Treatment of Nappy Rash

Treat any rash on your baby's bottom at the first sign, otherwise you may have a difficult job on your hands, and a secondary infection may set in through the weakened condition of the skin.

● Change nappies more frequently.

● Leave the nappy off in the fresh air and sunlight as much as possible.

● At each change, wash the skin with dilute herbal infusions or distilled *witch hazel*, dry it thoroughly and apply *marigold, camomile, chickweed* or *comfrey cream* to protect and heal it. If you suspect an infection, *marigold* and *camomile cream* will be beneficial as they are antiseptic.

● If you use fabric nappies, make sure they are sterilized properly and rinsed thoroughly so

that no bacteria or detergent is left to irritate the skin.

● Use one-way fabric nappy liners, which are designed to let the urine pass through to the nappy and leave the skin dry.

● Avoid plastic pants; use environmentally friendly, unbleached, disposable nappies for a while.

● Check inside your baby's mouth for white patches on the cheeks or tongue, which may indicate a thrush infection. If you wipe them away and they leave red patches underneath, your baby has oral thrush, which may have spread through the system to the anus, causing nappy rash. (To treat thrush see page 74.) Use a couple of drops of *marigold tincture* and *thyme* or *oregano oil* (1 drop for each 20ml tincture) in the mouth two or three times a day, or wipe a little plain live yoghurt round the mouth with your finger. Apply yoghurt, *marigold cream* or powdered *golden seal* to the bottom, after washing it with either dilute cider vinegar or *thyme* infusion.

● Egg white and oxygen is an old and very effective remedy for nappy rash. Apply egg white repeatedly to the affected area before putting on a nappy, and in between each application dry the bottom with a hair dryer. By doing this, you build up a thick protective layer of albumen, which can allow the skin to heal rapidly.

If the nappy rash is particularly bad, with spots, raised red patches, which may develop into red raw areas, or even shallow ulcers, your baby will feel very uncomfortable when he passes urine or a stool. To comfort him give *camomile tea* in between feeds, and apply soothing comfrey or *marshmallow ointment* alternated with more antiseptic *marigold* or *camomile cream*. Wash the bottom with infusions of *marigold, lavender, rosemary* or *elderflowers* or dilute *tincture of myrrh* or *marigold*.

CRADLE CAP

A thick, yellow-brown encrustation on a baby's scalp is cradle cap. Yellowish scales can appear in patches, especially on the top of the head, or they can cover the whole scalp. It can last until the child is three years old. It is a seborrhoeic condition, caused by over-activity of the glands in the skin that secrete sebum, and it is often associated with seborrhoeic dermatitis, a skin condition characterized by red, scaly areas, very often found on the forehead and eyebrows, as well as on the ears, behind the ears and in the fold of the thighs.

Because cradle cap occurs in babies who tend to have a greasy skin, it has nothing to do with cleanliness or hygiene as many suspect. Do not wash your baby's hair over-frequently or with soap, because this can make it worse. It is best to leave it alone if you are not worried about how it looks, and wait until the baby's tendency to produce more sebum settles down.

Treatment of Cradle Cap

• If you do want to clear it up, you can rub the scalp regularly with *olive oil*, mixed with a few drops of essential oil of *lavender, rosemary* or *lemon*, before putting your baby to bed, and wash off the loosened crusts with shampoo the following morning. You could also use *wheatgerm oil* or *St John's wort oil* with a few drops of *lavender oil* (use 1 teaspoon (5ml) base oil to 2 drops essential oil).

• To rinse the hair after shampooing you can use *heartsease, meadowsweet* or *burdock* infusion, or even common tea.

• Any loose flaky areas can be easily removed with a brush or a comb or a (clean) fingernail. But never pick off crusts that have not been loosened first, as it may cause bleeding, inflammation or infection of the scalp.

SEBORRHOEA

Over-production of sebum, causing cradle cap or seborrhoeic dermatitis, with red scaly areas on the face, on or behind the ears, and around the skin creases at the top of the thighs, frequently occurs in small babies.

Treatment of Seborrhoea

Seborrhoea often settles down of its own accord. If it does not, there are several things you can do to clear it quickly.

• It is often related to an allergic reaction, most commonly to milk products. If you are bottle-feeding it may be the cow's milk based formula that is the culprit, and it is worth investigating alternatives, such as soya milk or, if the baby is old enough, goat's milk or almond milk. If you are breast-feeding, it may be necessary for you to avoid eating all milk products – milk, cheese, cream, yoghurt, ice-cream – and all foods containing them for a period of time.

• If you are breast-feeding, eat plenty of other calcium-containing foods such as sesame seeds, dried figs, parsley, and watercress and nettle soup. Drink plenty of almond milk instead of cow's milk, and make sure that you eat enough foods containing magnesium and vitamin B6.

Almond Milk
Soak 1oz (25g) of freshly grated or ground almonds in 1 pint (600ml) of water for 24 hours. Stir well before drinking. Add any remaining sludge to your cereals or soups.

You should also take calcium-containing herbs, such as *comfrey, horsetail, kelp, marshmallow, meadowsweet, nettles* and *skullcap*, regularly in teas or tinctures. If your baby is on solids you can powder any of the above herbs and use ½ teaspoon (2–3ml) in cereal – use oat or millet flakes – once a day. Give *heartsease* and *meadowsweet tea* to drink three times a day, sweetening it with honey or unsweetened blackcurrant juice if you like.

• Apply *camomile cream* to the affected areas of the skin, or *St John's wort oil* with a little essential oil of *lavender*, two or three times a day until the skin clears.

• For breast-feeding mothers and babies, *burdock* decoction can be taken to help balance skin function and sebum production. You can take the normal therapeutic dose, flavoured with *peppermint* and/or *liquorice* if you like, and give the same tea, diluted in *fennel tea* in a ratio of one to three, between feeds.

COLIC

Colic is a kind of abdominal pain that comes and goes; it is caused by spasm of the gut. Some babies have what is called 'three-month colic', which describes the crying and apparent discomfort occurring mostly in the first twelve weeks of life. Other babies tend to cry more in the evenings and are said to have 'evening colic'. It is not always certain that the baby actually has colic, or even any abdominal pain, but it has been supposed that they have when they pass wind frequently – perhaps it is the crying that gives them the wind and they do not have colic at all. So it is not easy to be sure when your baby has colic, except when you have tried everything else to comfort them – feeding, changing, cuddling, walking up and down – or when they cry so much that their face goes red and both legs are drawn up to the stomach as if they are really in pain. This tends to occur after a feed, or in the evening when they are tired and their digestion does not function so efficiently. It is especially upsetting for mothers, when they feel they have tried everything and still the baby seems so distressed. Both need treatment!

• A baby's digestion is closely connected to their general sense of well-being and security, and this relates very much to their mother and how she is feeling. The more worried and tense you feel, often the more your baby will cry. If you feel yourself becoming stressed, it may be helpful to pass baby over for a little while to your partner or another member of the family while you try to relax a little on your own.

• Baby's colic can be caused by tension, but it can also be related to feeding problems, so it is important to check that the baby is latched on properly to the nipple and not gulping excessive air during the feed. This can often happen if your milk comes out too quickly at the beginning of a feed (you could express a little first by hand), or, if you are bottle-feeding, the hole in the teat may be too small or too big.

• It may also be that your baby is reacting allergically to a food substance coming through the breast milk, or that something in the milk is irritating the gut (as occurs in lactose intolerance), or that the formula milk does not suit them if they are being bottle-fed. Many colicky babies have been found to react to cow's milk in breast milk and formula milks. This is more likely in babies born of an allergic family in which problems such as eczema, asthma and hay fever occur. Other food substances coming through breast milk such as wheat, corn and citrus fruits, especially when they occur over frequently in the mother's diet, can also cause allergic reactions.

• Some other foods come through the breast milk and tend to cause colic or other digestive problems in babies:

☐ Curry or highly spiced foods can give tummy ache and diarrhoea
☐ Too much fruit – oranges, grapes, green apples, plums, strawberries, gooseberries, pineapple for example – can cause colic and diarrhoea
☐ Alcohol
☐ Coffee
☐ Onions, leeks, garlic
☐ Green peppers and aubergines
☐ Beans and lentils
☐ Cucumber
☐ Courgettes
☐ Brassicas (cabbage, cauliflower, brussel sprouts and so on)
☐ Chocolate
☐ Tomatoes
☐ Eggs
☐ Sugar

If any of these foods crop up regularly in your diet or you suspect them for any reason, omit one at a time completely from your diet for up to a week and note whether there is any improvement. To be sure, re-introduce the food after a week and watch for any reaction. This should enable you to determine which foods affect your baby's digestion, and then, when you start solid foods, be wary of foods that affected him and introduce these last of all, and only in small amounts at first.

Be careful not to compromise your own nutrition when you are breast-feeding. If you suspect one or several foods and you omit them from your diet, be careful to replace them with something else.

Treatment of Colic

● Before each feed give 1oz (30ml) of herbal tea to relax the gut and enhance the digestion. Choose from *angelica, camomile, caraway, catnip, cinnamon, dill, fennel, lemon balm* and *marshmallow*. Use $\frac{1}{4}$–$\frac{1}{2}$ teaspoon (2–3ml) of herbs to 4oz (100ml) boiling water. After the feed, if the baby seems uncomfortable or fretful give the tea again. *Slippery elm powder* mixed with warm water is often very soothing.

● You can use the same teas, but more concentrated, to add to bath water or to use as hand and foot baths. You can also drink stronger teas yourself, as the volatile oils from these herbs pass easily through the breast milk to the baby.

● If you or your baby seems particularly tense, add more relaxing herbs such as *catnip, limeflowers, camomile, lemon balm* or *hops* to the tea and bath for the baby; and *skullcap, vervain, passion flower, wild oats, lemon balm* or *camomile* for you.

● Essential oils can also be used. *Geranium, lavender, camomile, ginger, fennel* or *aniseed* can be diluted (2 drops to 1 teaspoon (5ml) base oil) and addded to bath water, used for massage or as compresses to the abdomen.

● Often, a warm bath with herbal infusions or essential oils will relax your baby beautifully before you feed, and you should find that feeding goes more smoothly.

● After a feed, when the baby is sleepy, try lying him on his side with a hot-water bottle wrapped in a towel close to his tummy. If he doesn't want to settle but doesn't want to suckle, it would be worth trying a dummy – it may work wonders!

If none of these measures proves effective and your baby is still crying over-frequently, seek specialist advice for diagnosis of possible medical problems or lactose intolerance.

VOMITING

If your baby regurgitates a little milk (known as possetting), this is nothing to worry about; it is quite normal and harmless. However:

● If your baby is less than ten weeks old and vomits forcefully (known as projectile vomiting) during or immediately after a feed, it could possibly mean pyloric stenosis. Consult your doctor.

● If you are giving your baby solid foods and he vomits during or after food, it may be that what he is eating does not agree with him, he is allergic to it, or the foods have not been pureed enough for him to digest.

● If your baby has a runny or blocked nose or a catarrhal cough, he may swallow mucus, which irritates the stomach and is brought back up often after coughing.

● If your baby seems unwell, off his food, flushed and irritable, or has watery stools, he may have an infection or mild gastro-enteritis.

If your baby is very distressed, in severe pain or passing stools that contain blood and mucus, contact your doctor immediately as the baby may have a blocked bowel.

Treatment of Vomiting

● It is important to replace any lost fluids if there is frequent vomiting during an infection, so make sure you offer the baby water, dilute juice or herbal teas mixed with honey frequently through the day. Reduce any fever with tepid sponging and appropriate herbs (see Fever, page 55).

● If your baby does not seem interested in feeding, express your milk so that your milk supply does not dwindle.

● To settle the stomach give weak herbal teas of either *camomile, catnip, cinnamon, dill, fennel, ginger, lemon balm* or *meadowsweet*, for example, sweetened with honey.

● If there are signs of infection, add *echinacea, elderflowers, limeflowers* or *thyme*. If there is accompanying diarrhoea, add *agrimony* or *tormentil*. Drinks or gruel made with *slippery elm powder*, a pinch of powdered *cinnamon* or *ginger*, mixed with warm water or expressed milk, can be very soothing to an upset stomach.

● You can also massage the abdomen or feet with dilute oils of *lemon balm (melissa)*, *lavender*, *peppermint* or *geranium* or apply compresses using these oils or the above infusions to the abdomen. Bath the baby in herbal water, using stronger infusions or dilute essential oils.

● If your baby has started to eat solids, give no solid food, just plenty of drink, until the stomach has settled down.

DIARRHOEA

Many babies have fairly loose stools, but as long as they are quite healthy and putting on weight, there is no cause for alarm.

● Diarrhoea can occur when a baby is teething, but it can also be related to food intolerance. Even when completely breast-fed, a baby may react to food substances, such as milk, wheat, corn, citrus fruits, coming through the milk. Formula milks can also be to blame. Once a baby starts solid food, food allergies can become more apparent, so if your baby develops diarrhoea when you introduce any new food, remove it from the diet and watch for any improvement. You may need to wait a few more months until the baby copes better with this food before introducing it again.

● Too much fruit, such as citrus fruits, green apples, strawberries and plums, dried fruit, such as apricots, figs or prunes, or fruit juice can also cause diarrhoea.

● If your baby seems unwell, irritable and flushed and has frequent, watery stools, it may be gastro-enteritis. This occurs far more frequently in bottle-fed babies than those who are breast-fed, as cow's milk formulae tend to produce more putrefactive bacteria in the bowel and do not protect a baby from infection in the same way as breast milk. Make sure that you give plenty of fluids – water or herbal teas – to guard against dehydration. Keep the baby off all solid foods until the bowels are back to normal, and then start with mushy brown rice and yoghurt, with a little honey and banana.

Treatment of Diarrhoea

● To help settle the stomach, add a little fresh lemon to water. Give herbal teas frequently through the day made from *blackberry leaf* and *raspberry leaf* with a pinch of *cinnamon*, or from *camomile, fennel, ginger, meadowsweet, peppermint* or *tormentil*.

● You can make a drink for babies who are old enough for solids from ½ cup live yoghurt, ½ cup boiled water, 1 teaspoon (5ml) grated *ginger* (fresh) and a pinch of *nutmeg*.

● *Slippery elm powder* with a pinch of *ginger* or *cinnamon powder*, made into a drink with a little warm water, is soothing to an irritated gut. *Arrowroot* is also useful to help stop diarrhoea.

● It may be that your baby's diarrhoea is related to tension. If you feel tense and worried, this may affect your baby, whose digestion will be affected. If you feel this may be a factor, try to relax when you are feeding, and use calming herbs – *lavender, camomile, limeflowers, catnip* or *lemon balm* – for yourself and your baby.

If acute, frequent diarrhoea persists in a baby for more than 24 hours, call your doctor.

CONSTIPATION

Constipation can affect both breast-fed and bottle-fed babies, although it tends to occur more in bottle-fed babies, whose bowels tend to breed more putrefactive bacteria. When it occurs in a breast-fed baby it is worth examining your own diet for food substances that may be irritating your baby's gut or producing an allergic reaction. Milk and wheat tend to be the most common culprits. Remove any foods you suspect for a week or two and see if the constipation improves.

When constipation occurs in bottle-fed babies, it is probable that the putrefactive bacteria in the gut are inhibiting the beneficial ones that enhance peristalsis, and that the more alkaline stools encourage the proliferation of pathogenic bacteria, which may irritate the gut, causing a degree of spasm.

In babies on solid food, it is possible that constipation can be caused by a number of factors:

• A low-fibre diet with too much refined food and sugar

• Too much animal protein from meat and dairy produce

• Not enough fluid intake

• Poor diet causing a deficiency of vitamins and minerals, particularly vitamin C and magnesium

• Anaemia

Treatment of Constipation

• Offer both breast-fed and bottle-fed babies more fluid between feeds, such as water, dilute fruit juices, water from cooked prunes, figs, raisins or apricots, or herbal teas: *camomile, fennel, ginger, lemon balm, peppermint* and *wild yam* will all help release tension or spasm in the gut, while *marshmallow* or *slippery elm powder* will soothe an irritated gut lining.

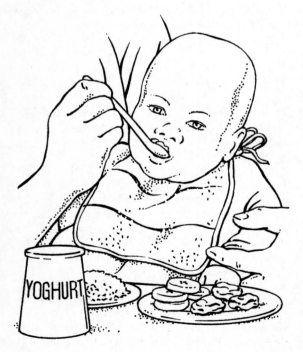

• Add a little *liquorice water* to herbal teas for a more laxative effect if necessary. Alternatively, try adding a little molasses (1 teaspoon to a cup of tea or hot water). Honey added to hot water or herbal tea also has a slightly laxative effect.

• Give babies on solid food mashed prunes and apricots – they will probably love them. Add desiccated coconut to cereals such as flaked rice, and try them with a little tahini. Give plain natural yoghurt with a little mashed banana to help re-establish the proper bacterial population of the gut. Try molasses in water and *slippery elm* gruel as well as the above herbal teas. Add *garlic* to their vegetables, and unrefined vegetable oils to their meals.

• You can also use essential oils for the baby's constipation. Try massaging the abdomen gently with a dilute oil of *ginger, cinnamon, camomile* or *fennel*, always in a clockwise direction (the same way as the bowel movements), or you could make the problem worse. Hot compresses applied to the abdomen can also be effective.

ALLERGIES

If you have a baby who is difficult, who cries or even yells a lot for no apparent reason, who has difficulty feeding or digesting, who suffers from colic, constipation, intermittent or frequent diarrhoea, or problems such as eczema, urticaria, nappy rash or other rashes, or constant colds, coughs or catarrh, this may well be the sign of an allergic reaction.

Allergic Symptoms

Allergic symptoms can be acute – diarrhoea and vomiting, colic or crying incessantly, for instance – or they may be vague. They could include irritability, sleeplessness, constant apparent hunger, congestion with mucus, dry skin or frequent possetting. There need not necessarily be an immediate reaction after food. If there is a family history of allergy, this is most likely to be the cause of these symptoms.

Treating an Allergic Baby

• If your baby is being breast-fed, it is likely that he is reacting to something you are eating, such as milk produce, wheat, eggs or citrus fruits. Exclude those foods you suspect or eat a lot of for two or three weeks and observe your baby's response. Many women worry about excluding milk produce from their diets, believing milk to be necessary to produce breast milk in adequate supply, and because of the relationship between calcium and the development of good tooth and bone structure. However, there are cultures in the world whose diets do not include milk produce and whose health does not seem to be compromised. Make sure that you eat plenty of calcium-containing foods from other sources on a regular basis instead (see page 177).

• Once an improvement is seen, you can try re-introducing foods slowly, one by one, with five days in between each new food, leaving cow's milk produce until last. Try small amounts initially, gradually increasing the amount if there is no adverse reaction. If the symptoms return, exclude them again and do not try them again for a month or two, after which your baby's digestion and immune system may be more mature and better able to cope.

• Bottle-fed babies who develop allergic symptoms may well be reacting to their formula feed. It is worth changing the formula to a soya-based milk and, once your baby is on solids, trying almond milk, goat's or sheep's milk instead.

• If you are breast-feeding it is worthwhile treating yourself. Follow the advice under How to Boost Immunity, page 70, and take recommended vitamins and mineral supplements, essential fatty acids and herbal remedies, as these will be passed through the milk to treat your baby.

• Give your baby dilute herbal teas made from *camomile, fennel, marshmallow, wild yam* or *yarrow* to aid digestion and soothe the allergic response.

• Providing there is no diarrhoea, you can flavour the teas with a little *liquorice*; otherwise use honey.

• *Slippery elm gruel* (see page 135) is also recommended.

• Dilute essential oils can be used to reduce the allergic response and to modify the over-reaction of the immune system. *Camomile, lavender* and *melissa (lemon balm)* are the most successful for treating allergies. Add 2 drops to (5ml) base oil and use it in the bath, for massaging your baby, or for heating in a vaporizer in the bedroom. *Camomile* is particularly useful for skin irritation.

• Breast milk is the best food for a baby born of allergic parents or relations. The longer you can breast-feed, the better protected your baby will be. Do not try to wean too early or to introduce solid foods before six months. Leave the foods that are likely to cause problems – wheat, milk, eggs and citrus fruits, or any other foods that you or your partner are allergic to – until your baby is over a year old.

• Try to avoid your baby being in contact with toxins that may exacerbate the problem. Cigarette smoke is particularly bad for babies prone to colds, coughs, catarrh and frequent upper respiratory infections. Chemicals in tap water should be avoided, so use bottled water as far as you can. Check the effects of any drugs you may be taking, and try not to give your baby antibiotics, as candidiasis (see page 73) could really add to your baby's problems. Keep away from foods with artificial colourings, flavourings and preservatives, and buy organic foods where you can.

STICKY EYE

This mild infection of the eyes causes a yellowish discharge and crusting on the eyelids and lashes, and it is very common in the first week of life. It is usually due to a foreign substance perhaps a little amniotic fluid or blood, getting into the eye during the birth.

Treatment of Sticky Eye

• Use a weak infusion of *camomile, marigold, elderflower* or *marshmallow* (use boiled or distilled water for this) and wash both eyes with it when warm, using clean cotton wool for each eye. Always start at the outside corner of the eye and wipe downwards. You can also use a little breast milk, or a mixture of almond oil and *rose water* to wipe the eyelid, but be careful not to get the oil in the eye. A saline solution, made from 1 teaspoon of sea salt to 1 cup boiled water, can be very effective.

• Put your baby to sleep with the bad eye uppermost to let the air circulate round it and to prevent the other eye from being infected from the sheet. Change the bed clothes frequently.

SLEEPING PROBLEMS

One of the major upheavals in many parents' lives is the change in sleep patterns. Very often a woman is prepared for this during pregnancy when in the last few weeks she tends to wake up frequently during the night, a pattern that will tend to go on for several weeks, often months, once the baby is born.

The amount and pattern of sleep that a baby needs varies from one baby to another – some sleep for several hours at a stretch and can sleep through the night when just a few weeks old. Others are more wakeful and need to be fed every hour or two, even through the night, and some reverse a normal adult sleep pattern and sleep for long periods through the day and very little at night. Like all other animals whose young snuggle up to the mother to sleep, babies feel most happy, secure and relaxed near their mother, so that if you have a very wakeful baby, you may find if you carry her in a sling across your front she will get more sleep in the day and give you some space to do the things you want. At night you may find the best way for both of you to get the most sleep is to take the baby in bed with you so that you have hardly to stir when your baby wants to feed. Otherwise you may find that if you impose strict rules, such as sleeping in a separate cot or for a certain length of time you may well end up tired and frazzled, as you will find it hard to persuade a baby to sleep when she doesn't want to. As every parent who has had a wakeful baby must know, it is very hard to maintain the often necessary level of functioning when you are trying to manage on very little sleep.

When you put a young baby in a cot you will probably find that, if you wrap her firmly and snugly in a sheet or shawl and then tuck something over her, she will feel more secure and sleep longer. If she wakes, it is usually for a feed and for reassurance. As the baby gets older, she will probably not want to be so restricted and will have longer periods awake, looking around and wanting to play.

It is important to understand that adults and babies do not have the same sleep patterns. Do not expect your baby to sleep in an adult fashion and then get frustrated or disappointed when this does not happen. Babies spend about half their sleeping time in a light sleep, known as rapid eye movement (REM) sleep, when they are dreaming. Because of this, it is quite normal for a baby or toddler to wake up several times in the night. When your baby does wake, feed and cuddle her, but discourage play by putting her in the cot or next to you in bed and close your eyes and try to go to sleep – this will help your baby to get back to sleep, too.

Treatment for Sleeping Problems

For remedies for aiding sleep see Crying Baby, page 56 and Insomnia, page 127.

If you have a very wakeful baby, and none of the above suggestions seem to work for you, it may be that there are other reasons for your baby's restlessness and insomnia. It could be related to teething, colic, an infection, an itchy skin, being too hot or not warm enough, a snuffly nose or a sore bottom. Hyperactivity may also be a problem (see page 126).

TEETHING

Babies normally teeth from five or six months onwards, and they often produce teeth with no trouble at all.

Teething Symptoms

Some babies tend to dribble a lot when teething; others may develop rashes on the face, become irritable, clingy and restless, go off their food or have trouble sleeping. It may be that this predisposes them to many of the other symptoms that are associated with teething, such as fever, diarrhoea, generalized rashes, colds and other infections and rubbing their ears. Nevertheless, these may have absolutely nothing to do with teething and should always be checked out as symptoms indicating other illness or imbalance.

So, if your baby is dribbling and goes off his food, check his gums. They may look red and swollen and there may even be a blister on the gum overlying the tooth coming through.

Treatment for Teething Problems

• If there are blisters on the gum, give your baby something to chew on – either your finger, hopefully not your nipple, *a marshmallow root* or *liquorice stick* or a teething ring – you could cool this in the fridge for a while for extra relief.

• You can also rub the gums, try a little honey, or honey with a drop of *camomile oil* or *clove oil*.

• Give infusions of either *camomile, limeflowers, yarrow, fennel* or *catnip* frequently through the day.

FEVERS

If your baby is off his food, seems fretful or irritable and looks a little flushed, it is as well to check the temperature – this needs to be done rectally (see page 84). The temperature-regulating mechanisms of babies and children are less effective than those of adults, and so fevers can develop easily in babies and temperatures can swing up and down in quick succession, tending to be higher in the afternoon or evening.

If your baby has a fever, it probably indicates the onset of an infection – a cold, sore throat, or a tummy bug, perhaps – so you need to keep an eye on any associated symptoms or developments. Since a fever represents the body's fight against infection, it is a healthy reaction and not something that needs to be suppressed unless it is high.

Treatment for Fever

• If the baby feels very hot, and the temperature is over 100°F (38°C) remove the clothes

and just leave a vest and nappy on. If the baby is in a cot, just cover with a sheet. Make sure the room is not too hot or too cold, and that the baby is not in a draught, but that there is plenty of fresh air in the room.

• Offer plenty of fluids to prevent dehydration – both the breast and dilute juice, water and herbal teas. *Camomile, catnip, elderflower, limeflowers* and *yarrow* will increase perspiration and help to bring the fever down. Their volatile oils also have antiseptic properties. Use the same infusions for *tepid* sponging. Make sure you do not use cold water, as this will reduce heat loss via the skin by closing up the pores. You can also use these infusions in the bath, or use a few drops of essential oil of *peppermint, lavender* or *eucalyptus* in bath water and for tepid sponging. Use these essential oils in a vaporizer in the room as this will also help enhance the body's fight against the infection.

• Alternatively, you could apply compresses to the baby's body, head, abdomen or feet using these infusions and essential oils. You can leave a flannel soaked in these around the feet for a while, when the baby is asleep.

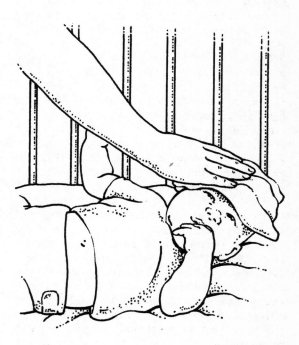

• If your baby seems particularly restless and cannot settle, use predominantly *limeflower* and *camomile* tea, and essential oils of *camomile* or *lavender*. If you can get the baby to sleep, this is the most healing thing of all and will probably mean that whatever heralded the fever is resolved in no time.

If a fever persists over 24 hours or if you are worried about any accompanying symptoms, consult your practitioner.

For more detailed discussion of fevers and their treatment see pages 82–88; for specific infections and their treatment, see the appropriate sections in Childrens' Ailments.

A CRYING BABY

All babies cry; it is normally their way of telling you they are hungry. Some babies cry more than others. If your baby is breast-fed he or she may cry more than a bottle-fed baby because breast milk tends to pass through the stomach quite quickly, so the baby may get hungry frequently through the day and night. Most healthy babies stop crying as soon as they are being fed and cuddled, or made comfortable through a change of nappy. Sometimes, your baby will still cry – very often in the evenings, if your milk supply is dwindling, or perhaps if he or she has 'evening *colic*' (see page 49).

You will soon learn to recognize what your baby means when he or she cries – whether he is just hungry and wants to be picked up, feels restless or uncomfortable, is irritable because he wants to sleep, or is just bored. You will probably be able to tell if it is colic as the cry will be more distressed, or if he does not feel well as the cry will vary from the normal pattern and could go on intermittently through the day. This could mean *teething*, so check the gums and observe whether he is dribbling a lot (see page 54). It could also mean an infection is developing; take the temperature or call your practitioner if you need to. After a day or so you may see symptoms, such as a runny nose or cough, or a common childhood infection come out. Then you can treat accordingly (see Childrens' Ailments).

Treatment to Calm a Crying Baby

You can use herbs to calm your baby and encourage a restful sleep for your baby, and, of course, for yourself.

Warm Herbal Baths When you bathe the baby, add strong infusions of relaxing herbs: Choose from *camomile, catnip, cowslip, hops, lavender, lemon balm* and *limeflowers*. Dilute essential oils can be used in bath water; *camomile, geranium, lavender, neroli* and *rose* are all very helpful. The warmth of the bath is relaxing in itself, and the addition of herbs will help to induce calm, releasing tension in muscles and in the gut, and soothing discomfort related to fevers or skin problems. If your baby seems to wake from sleep in a distressed state, *catnip* is particularly recommended.

Massage When you put your baby to bed, if he or she still seems restless, massage the feet or abdomen, or stroke the head with some dilute essential oils, until he or she drops off, or rock the cradle and use the oils in a vaporizer near the bed.

Herbal Teas Dilute teas of the above herbs can also be given before bed, on a spoon or in a bottle and repeated if the baby wakes and cannot get back to sleep easily.

Bach Remedies Bach Flower Remedies often work well with distress, crying or sleeping problems, especially when they are related to insecurity, fear and not wanting to be left alone (see page 165).

It is easier to comfort a crying baby if you know what the trouble is, but what is hardest for most parents is when the baby cries and nothing you do seems to make a jot of difference. You will probably hear stories from friends and relations of walking up and down the room for hours on end, rhythmically rocking the baby, or going out in the car in the middle of the night to get the baby to sleep after all else has failed, and you may find yourself doing the same. Often a baby responds better to noisy and fast motion as in a car or pram, rather than quiet and gentle rocking in a cot. Many babies stop crying if you talk to them and show them things and get them interested in something, instead of trying to relax them into sleep.

When you have a crying baby you may be offered a wealth of advice, often conflicting, about what you can do to comfort him or her. Some may try to persuade you to leave your baby crying as it is 'good for her' or 'it never does to spoil them' or 'it can't be time for her feed yet'. It may be hard for you to find your own way through this, but you will probably find that if you give your baby what he or she needs and respond to every cry for help, that he or she will be generally more contented and secure, even if there are some crying times.

Treatment for the Mother of a Crying Baby

Of course, a crying baby can have a profound effect on a mother's feelings. You may feel either anxiety, panic, pure frustration and then relief when the crying stops. You may feel very distressed and at the end of your tether. It is important at this point to take a break. If possible, ask someone else to hold your baby for a while – you never know, this may just do the trick. The baby may have sensed your tension or frustration. The Bach Flower Remedies are very useful; *Rescue Remedy* would be quite appropriate here (see page 167). Remember that it is quite normal for a mother to feel concerned or even distressed if her baby cries; nature has designed things so that the powerful connection between mother and offspring will ensure that the baby is nurtured until it is more able to look after him or herself, and a signal such as crying cannot be ignored. It may be that sometimes you have to give up other activities or plans, just to be with your baby, let go of ideas of how you want things to be or how they should be, and be there for him or her.

If you feel that your baby's crying may indicate an underlying medical condition, trust your feelings and consult your practitioner or ask for specialist advice.

PART III
HERBAL CHILD CARE

CHAPTER 7

THE IMMUNE SYSTEM

UNDERSTANDING THE IMMUNE SYSTEM

An efficient immune system is the key to a robust and healthy child, who will be able to resist infections and allergy and who will get the most out of life without being hampered by illness. Our bodies' defences are so wonderfully designed that, despite the millions of potentially disease-producing organisms and substances – bacteria, viruses, fungi, parasites and allergens – that surround us, we survive, only occasionally falling prey to infection. When that happens, our immune systems should attack the invaders and set up healing and repair. As long as a child is basically healthy and well nourished, he or she will recover quickly and easily.

Among the intricate mechanisms our bodies possess to prevent the entry of micro-organisms are:

eyes	antiseptic tears
mouth	antiseptic saliva
nose	sticky mucus and hairs to trap organisms – sneezing expels them forcibly
chest	mucus and hairs (muco-ciliary escalator), trapping organisms and pollutants and preventing them invading the lungs – coughing expels them forcibly
stomach	acid destroys organisms
intestine	gut flora check unwanted organisms, and the bowels expel them and toxins
bladder	flushes out organisms and toxins through urine
vagina	acid destroys organisms
skin	waterproof, protects underlying tissues, secretes sebum and antiseptic oils.

Should any of these mechanisms be faulty or should microbes invade the tissues, the immune system rallies its defences to attack the pathogens in two different ways: one to deal with all types of invaders, the other with more specific responses to individual types of organisms.

When microbes invade the body – through a cut on the skin, for example – an inflammatory process is set up, which is designed to repel the invasion and heal the damaged tissues. The tiny blood vessels in the area dilate to bring more blood to the area, including white blood cells to attack the bacteria. Cells around the wound release certain chemicals, including histamine, which attract the white blood cells to pass from the blood vessels into the damaged tissues. The blood vessels become more permeable, allowing plasma proteins to help in defence and repair of the tissues.

If the resulting inflammation, which is intentionally hot, red and swollen, does not clear the infection, back-up measures are put into motion. More powerful white blood cells (monocytes), which can attack and destroy more bacteria at once, move into the area. Should this not do the trick, the lymphatic system is rallied into action. This is a network of tiny vessels carrying lymph, a colourless fluid, which picks up debris and microbes, and carries it to the lymph nodes, where there are concentrations of white blood cells – some called macrophages, which engulf and eat up the microbes and filter the debris, and others

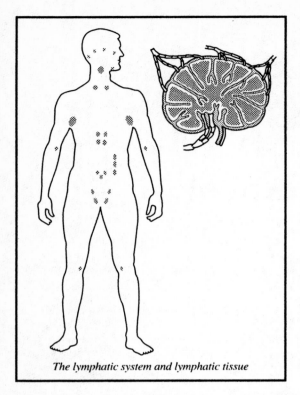

The lymphatic system and lymphatic tissue

called lymphocytes, which produce antibodies to the invading organisms. Some of these stay in the lymph nodes, while others travel, carried via the lymph. Lymph nodes occur in clusters along the main channels of the lymphatic system, especially around the ears and neck, the armpits, the groin (where they can be felt when swollen) and the chest and abdomen (where they cannot be felt). When the system is under attack, the lymph nodes enlarge as more lymphocytes are produced to go into battle — for example, when a child gets a sore throat the lymph nodes in the neck swell up and feel tender.

Children have other lymphatic tissue that plays an important part in the development of their immunity. The thymus gland, the home of the T-cells that attack infected cells, which is located at the junction of the neck and chest, is far larger in children than in adults; it gradually dwindles in size as the child's immunity becomes established. The spleen and liver, tonsils, adenoids and the wall of the small intestine all contain plenty of lymphatic tissue. Common infections that develop in childhood, such as chicken pox and German measles, often cause swelling and tenderness of lymphatic tissue, some generalized throughout the body, others more specifically affecting some glands — those around the ears and at the back of the neck in German measles, for instance.

Should these measures still not repel a highly infectious invasion, specific immune responses come into effect. Molecules on the surface of the infecting organisms (antigens) stimulate lymphocytes and produce antibodies to combine with each specific antigen. These antibodies have a memory, so that should the same infection recur, the antigens are recognized so rapidly that the body is able to deal effectively with the organisms in the lymphatic system and bloodstream before an infection develops.

B-cells and T-cells are the major classes of lymphocytes that are responsible for antibody production. T-cells mature in the thymus gland. Some deal with infections, such as viruses that get inside the body's cells. T-killer cells attack infected cells with a cell poison. Others, T-helper cells, communicate with B-cells and call them to battle, and T-suppressor cells control the action of other lymphocytes and stop it from getting out of hand, calling a halt to the attack once the infection is resolved. B-cells mature in the bone marrow and produce antibodies to bind to the specific antigens. Once they have done this, they multiply repeatedly into plasma cells, which manufacture the antibodies for the bloodstream, and B-memory cells, which rapidly provide immunity against that particular infection in the future.

Babies are born with very little immunity — only that which they inherit from their mothers (passive immunity), and which only lasts for their first year of life. Breast-feeding provides them with many of the raw materials to manufacture their own defences, and so provides a good start to establish their immune systems.

However, in order to produce specific antibodies to individual infections they need initially to be infected by each type of organism, and it is for this reason that small children tend to develop frequent infections. Children aged eight, nine or ten years tend to develop far fewer infections than those who are younger.

Once the bacteria and viruses have been destroyed by the immune system, the debris needs to be cleared from the system, and this is the work of the liver, to which the debris is carried. All food and toxins absorbed by the intestines are also taken to the liver, which has an intricate system of tiny blood vessels lined with white blood cells that destroy unwanted matter brought to the liver via the bloodstream. Other matter is brought to the liver – dead cells, hormones, toxins, drugs, and substances such as pesticides and food additives – which are rendered harmless by various enzymatic reactions. The liver is a competent detoxifying organ, which has to work hard in our polluted world, and its efficient functioning is vital to the maintenance of a healthy immune system. It processes the nutrients absorbed from the digestive tract, which not only provide the raw materials for the immune system, but also for healing and repair. If the liver is struggling under too great a burden of toxins, it will not be able to respond efficiently when the body is invaded by infectious organisms.

THE RAW MATERIALS OF THE IMMUNE SYSTEM

Proteins

Not only are proteins vital to growth and repair, providing the basic building blocks of our bodies, but they are also vital for the normal function of the immune system by providing for formation of antibodies.

Chicken, fish, eggs and soya beans provide us with complete proteins, while other vegetable sources of protein – grains, nuts and seeds, beans and pulses – need to be combined in the same meal to provide all the essential amino acids.

Essential Fatty Acids

These are fats that cannot be made by the body; they have to be taken in the diet. Essential fatty acids (EFAs) are vital to a healthy immune system, and yet the average diet is very low in these and high in the kinds of fats that are harmful – a fact that is becoming increasingly clear through health education, especially in reference to heart disease. Not only do EFAs reduce cholesterol and protect against heart and arterial disease, but they are also crucial to the normal function of lymphocytes and their production of antibodies, to a healthy skin, blood and kidneys, to the formation of the membrane of every cell in the body as well as to the normal function of the brain and nervous system.

Essential Fatty Acids

Omega–6	Omega–3
seeds	linseed oil (food grade)
corn	soya beans, soya oil
evening primrose	walnuts, walnut oil
sunflower oil	wheat germ, wheat germ oil
safflower oil	fresh oily fish
grains	cod liver oil
vegetables	dried beans
dried beans	sprouted beans
sprouted seeds and beans	spinach and cabbage
	wheat

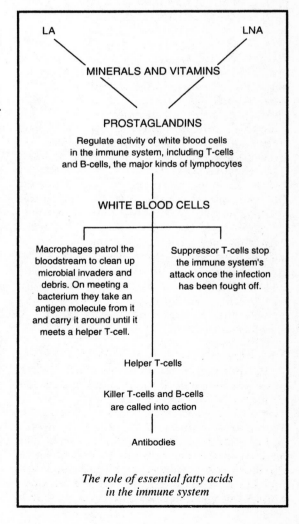

The role of essential fatty acids in the immune system

There are two main groups of EFAs: **omega–6** (the main ones being linoleic acid (LA) and arachidonic acid) and **omega–3** (the main one being linolenic acid (LNA)). Omega–6 EFAs are found mainly in seeds, such as safflower, sunflower, pumpkin, as well as corn and evening primrose, and the oils pressed from these. They are also found in grains and vegetables. Omega–3 EFAs are found in linseed oil, soya oil, walnut and wheat germ oil as well as in fresh wheat germ. All these oils need to be cold-pressed, fresh and unrefined; most commercial oils are heat-extracted, and heat damages the essential fatty acids. They are also chemically refined, bleached and hydrogenated, which destroys most of their nutritional value.

Omega–3 oils are also found in fresh oily fish, such as sardines, tuna, salmon, herring and mackerel, and in cod liver oil. Canning, processing and cooking can all destroy essential fatty acids. Green vegetables – cabbage and spinach, for example – and wheat are moderate sources. Both types of oils are found in dried beans, such as haricot and soya, and in sprouted beans, such as mung beans.

Once taken in through the diet, EFAs have to be converted into other forms through the child's metabolism before they can be used. The enzymes involved in their metabolism require other nutrients (vitamins A, C, E and B6) and minerals (zinc, copper, magnesium and selenium) to process them into prostaglandins, hormone-like substances that have a variety of roles including affecting the immune system. One type of prostaglandin, E1, stimulates T-suppressor lymphocytes, which stop abnormal cells from multiplying and white blood cells from attacking the body's own tissues, and if these do not work efficiently, allergies and auto-immune disease will result.

Vitamins, Minerals and Trace Elements

A variety of vitamins, minerals and trace elements are essential to the immune system and EFA metabolism.

Vitamin A Crucial to the production of T and B white blood cells, which are responsible for the production of antibodies. Vitamin A deficiency will mean that the body is not able to produce enough antibodies to ward off infection. A serious deficiency can cause atrophy of the lymphatic tissue in the thymus gland and spleen, thus severely reducing resistance to infection.

B Vitamins The most important of these is vitamin B6, but they are all vital to the healthy functioning of the mucous membranes and a first line of defence against micro-organisms, as well as being crucial in the production of T and B white blood cells and the formation of antibodies. Vitamin B6 needs zinc in order to be fully effective.

Vitamin C This helps to protect against virus infections, it stimulates the large white blood cells (macrophages), which eat up invading micro-organisms, and it encourages antibody response and the production of T-killer cells. Vitamin C also reduces the effects of many allergic reactions, as well as the immuno-suppressive effects of stress through its effect on the adrenal glands.

Vitamin E This enhances the production of antibodies and the activity of macrophages, and the body's resistance, particularly to viruses. It works even better together with selenium. Like vitamins A and C, it is a powerful anti-oxidant, reducing the cell damage caused when oxygen combines with other substances, and it helps to prevent damage to the lungs caused by pollution in the atmosphere. Anti-oxidants are vital for the immune system, helping to protect the white blood cells from destroying themselves in the battle against infection, which gives off a lot of heat.

Copper This is necessary for a child's resistance to infection, but too much can actually suppress the immune system.

Iron T-cells and B-cells need plenty of oxygen, and because iron-containing haemoglobin carries the oxygen in the bloodstream, the immune system requires a good supply of iron. However, excess iron can actually be harmful, because micro-organisms need iron to be able to multiply.

Magnesium The metabolism of EFA into prostaglandin requires magnesium, which, when balanced with calcium, is particularly responsible for the normal relaxation of the muscular system. The over-use of artificial fertilizers and

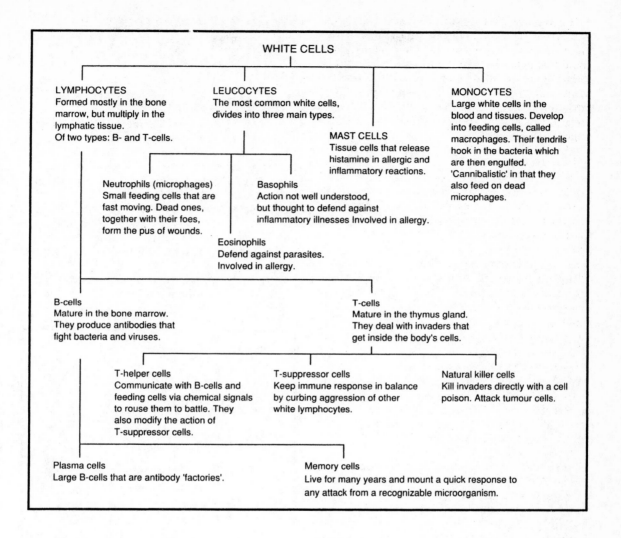

WHITE CELLS

LYMPHOCYTES
Formed mostly in the bone
marrow, but multiply in the
lymphatic tissue.
Of two types: B- and T-cells.

LEUCOCYTES
The most common white cells,
divides into three main types.

MONOCYTES
Large white cells in the
blood and tissues. Develop
into feeding cells, called
macrophages. Their tendrils
hook in the bacteria which
are then engulfed.
'Cannibalistic' in that they
also feed on dead
microphages.

MAST CELLS
Tissue cells that release
histamine in allergic and
inflammatory reactions.

Neutrophils (microphages)
Small feeding cells that are
fast moving. Dead ones,
together with their foes,
form the pus of wounds.

Basophils
Action not well understood,
but thought to defend against
inflammatory illnesses Involved in allergy.

Eosinophils
Defend against parasites.
Involved in allergy.

B-cells
Mature in the bone marrow.
They produce antibodies that
fight bacteria and viruses.

T-cells
Mature in the thymus gland.
They deal with invaders that
get inside the body's cells.

T-helper cells
Communicate with B-cells and
feeding cells via chemical signals
to rouse them to battle. They
also modify the action of
T-suppressor cells.

T-suppressor cells
Keep immune response in balance
by curbing aggression of other
white lymphocytes.

Natural killer cells
Kill invaders directly with a cell
poison. Attack tumour cells.

Plasma cells
Large B-cells that are antibody 'factories'.

Memory cells
Live for many years and mount a quick response to
any attack from a recognizable microorganism.

phosphorus in preserved foods has meant that magnesium can be deficient in diets that have a predominance of refined or junk foods or that contain excess bran, which binds magnesium and makes it unavailable to the body.

Selenium This enhances the immune system, particularly the activity of the macrophages and antibodies. It is another powerful anti-oxidant and helps the body to eliminate heavy, immuno-suppressive metals such as mercury, cadmium and lead.

Zinc In association with vitamin B6, zinc is the most vital mineral to the efficient working of the immune system, being involved particularly in the production of T-cells and in healing and repair. The average diet tends to be deficient in both selenium and zinc, because poor soil and the overuse of artificial fertilizers produces foods low in these substances. Zinc deficiency is common among young children who derive a lot of their nutrition from milk and cheese.

For more information about, and food sources of, the above nutrients see Diet Chart, page 173.

The best way to ensure that your children have sufficient of these nutrients is to give them a diet that is high in fresh, organically grown foods, with as much fresh fruit and vegetables as possible, but that is low in saturated fats. It should also be high in grains, nuts, seeds, beans

65

and pulses, oily fish and cold-pressed vegetable oils. Refined foods, packet, tinned and frozen foods, excess sugar and salt, fatty meats, dairy produce, cakes, biscuits and sweets should be avoided. Many of these are actually classed as 'anti-nutrients' – that is, they either have very little nutritional value or they disturb EFA metabolism and, therefore, adversely affect the immune system.

Foods to be Avoided

Sugar   Excessive amounts of sugar are harmful to the metabolism of EFAs and rob the body of B vitamins and minerals, particularly magnesium and copper, which are vital to the immune system.

Salt   Too much salt, which is particularly found in processed foods, upsets the sodium/magnesium/potassium balance in the body and leads to a loss of magnesium and potassium.

Saturated Fats and Refined Oils   Excessive quantities of saturated fats and refined oils interfere with the body's ability to use EFAs; partially hydrogenated vegetable oils are the worst culprits. The enzymes that process EFAs use these other fats instead, mistaking them for the real thing, but the immune system is unable to use them in the same way.

Preserved, Processed Foods and Fizzy Drinks   These often contain large amounts of phosphates, which interfere with the absorption of nutrients, such as magnesium and calcium, from the digestive tract. Pesticide residues in food inhibit the body's use of vitamin B6 and increase the body's need for anti-oxidants.

Fried Food   When oils are heated, especially by those who keep oil hot all day or repeatedly re-use the same oil to deep fry fish, chicken and chips, chemicals called free radicals are created. These can damage cell membranes and EFAs. Anti-oxidants help prevent such damage, and their defence system involves a number of nutrients, including vitamins A, C, B and E and zinc, copper, sulphur and magnesium. Heated oils, pesticides in food and environmental pollutants obviously increase the body's need for these nutrients, and their use in this way prevents them from being available to the same extent to the immune system.

HOW THE IMMUNE SYSTEM CAN GO WRONG (WHY DO CHILDREN GET ILL?)

INFECTIONS

When certain germs penetrate the body's outer defences and invade the tissues, there begins a race to see which can multiply faster – the infecting organisms or the B-cells producing antibodies. If a child is healthy, the B-cells should win, but if it is a particularly strong infection or one that the child's body has not encountered before – the first exposure to chicken pox, mumps or measles, for example – or the immune system is impaired, the germs will win.

Although drugs and vaccinations have reduced the incidence and severity of several

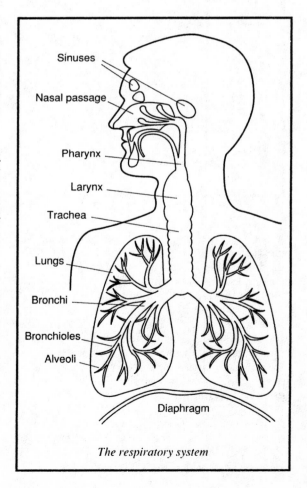

The respiratory system

acute childhood illnesses, such as scarlet fever, diphtheria, polio and whooping cough, chronic infections and allergies are rapidly on the increase. The incidence of asthma and hay fever has almost doubled in the last few years, and allergic skin conditions are fast following suit.

ALLERGIES

When the immune system rallies its defences against substances that are not infectious or harmful but that may actually be useful and nutritious, this is known as allergy. When it attacks the body's own tissues, it is known as auto-immune disease, which is unusual in chil-

---

Common Allergens Causing Allergic Reactions

External
animal dander
dust mites
drugs such as
  penicillin
pollens
spores from moulds
household
  chemicals
plants – primulas,
  for example
environmental
  pollutants
biological washing
  powders
creams and
  ointments
wool
sunlight
insect venoms

Internal
cow's milk
  products and beef
goat's and sheep's
  milk products
wheat
food additives –
  colourings,
  flavourings and
  preservatives
foods with
  chemical residues
  – pesticides,
  fungicides and so
  on
meat products
  containing
  antibiotic or
  steroid residues
shellfish
eggs
oranges
strawberries
tomatoes
chocolate
pork
sugar

Symptoms of Allergic Reactions

An allergic reaction represents the body's effort to rid itself of something it interprets as harmful – bacteria, a virus or a foreign body, for instance. It varies from one susceptible child to another and could arise as any of the following:

- [ ] asthma
- [ ] eczema
- [ ] urticaria
- [ ] dry or rough skin
- [ ] chronic catarrh or sinusitis
- [ ] hay fever or allergic rhinitis
- [ ] frequent respiratory infections – colds, coughs, tonsilitis, ear infections or glue ear
- [ ] coeliac disease and malabsorption
- [ ] chronic constipation or diarrhoea and colic
- [ ] tiredness and malaise
- [ ] conjunctivitis
- [ ] behavioural problems and hyperactivity, temper tantrums and poor concentration, learning problems
- [ ] insomnia, poor sleep patterns
- [ ] convulsions, continual thirst, bedwetting
- [ ] low blood sugar
- [ ] food cravings
- [ ] muscle or joint pains, aching legs
- [ ] headaches
- [ ] fussy eating

---

dren, although it is becoming increasingly prevalent among adolescents and young adults – for example, Crohn's disease and ulcerative colitis.

An allergic reaction involves an exaggerated immune response to a variety of substances, which may be natural or artificial, foods or other chemical substances, including proteins such as pollen, which causes hay fever, or the house-dust mite, which is involved in asthma.

The symptoms produced in many allergic responses are related to the release of chemicals such as histamine. Lining the mucous membranes, such as those in the respiratory and intestinal tracts, are white blood cells, similar to B-cells and known as mast-cells, which produce special antibodies known as immuno-globulins, and these have a memory. When an allergic reaction occurs, immunoglobulins are formed, and they bind to mast-cells, ready to form a complex with the allergen when the person is exposed to the same substance again, and attach to the surface of various cells in blood-vessels and tissues. When this occurs, histamine and other chemicals and prostaglan-dins are released, causing symptoms, such as the inflammation of the nasal passages, over-production of mucus and irritation of the eyes that characterize hay fever; inflammation of the digestive tract producing diarrhoea; asthma; and urticaria.

The term 'atopy' implies a susceptibility to develop immediate allergies on exposure to certain substances, such as atopic eczema, asthma and hay fever.

Different Ways of Contact

By mouth Babies and children often react allergically to foods or drugs. Milk, eggs, wheat, shellfish and strawberries are common culprits, and penicillin often causes a drug reaction. Symptoms can vary widely, ranging from swelling of the face, stomach aches, vomiting and diarrhoea to urticaria or hives, wheezing and even anaphylactic shock, causing circulatory collapse and extreme distress. Some children have very specific allergies – for exam-ple, only to shellfish or only to tomatoes – and some react only to large amounts of the incri-minated food, while others require just a few molecules to set the wheels of the allergic res-ponse in motion.

Through the Nose Some children react to substances that are inhaled. Household chemi-cals, environmental pollutants, pollens, dust, animal dander and moulds can lead to res-ponses such as itching or swollen eyes, sneez-ing, runny nose, chronic catarrh, congestion of the throat or chest, coughing and wheezing, and even eczema, which is common in the hay fever season.

Through the Skin Many environmental substances and common household chemicals can cause skin rashes on contact – biological washing powders, for example, leave residues

in the clothes and these enzymes start to break down the proteins in the skin. Wool, various plants, bases, creams and ointments (such as lanolin), strong sunlight and extreme cold can also trigger an allergic response.

Allergic responses may also vary according to age. Broadly speaking, babies react to skin con-tact and what they eat, toddlers to the same as well as what they become infected by, and older children react to all of these and also to what they inhale.

Allergies in Babies

Babies have very delicate skins, which can react to wool, baby lotions and ointments, nylon, rubber pants, disposable nappies and washing powder. Their immature digestive tracts can react to foods, such as formula milks, but also to substances that come through breast milk including milk produce, wheat, eggs and drugs.

If you suspect that your baby has an allergy, think back over your pregnancy for symptoms that might constitute an allergic response. This may give you some clues as to which allergens your baby may be reacting to – for example, particularly bad morning sickness, rhinitis or catarrh, or bowel problems may suggest imbal-ance of wheat or milk. Babies of allergic parents are more likely to react allergically, and often to similar substances, than those of parents with no positive history of allergy.

Symptoms of Allergy in a Baby

- ☐ A baby who cries or yells a lot – 'a difficult baby'
- ☐ Feeding difficulties or colic
- ☐ Constipation or diarrhoea
- ☐ Eczema, urticaria, prickly heat or other rashes
- ☐ Dry skin or persistent nappy rash
- ☐ Insomnia and irritability
- ☐ Constant apparent hunger
- ☐ Frequent possetting
- ☐ Congestion with mucus – leading to problems such as bronchiolitis and croup and frequent respiratory infections

Allergies in Toddlers

Many toddlers develop frequent colds, bronchiolitis, croup, chest infections or ear infections, and they may also be given antibiotics, which serve only to exacerbate the problem, putting further stress on the immune system. Often the mother had similar symptoms during pregnancy – frequent colds or coughs, sore throats or catarrh, for instance – and in many cases these women drank a lot of milk for its calcium content. Milk produce is most often the culprit in these cases. The incidence of respiratory infections can reduce dramatically if milk produce is reduced or omitted from the diet.

Allergies in Older Children

As children get older, they tend to develop the same allergic symptoms as adults, and they may well begin to follow the same pattern as allergic parents or close relatives – hay fever, asthma, bowel problems, chronic eczema, headaches or migraines, for example.

Children who had allergies as a baby or toddler, may well 'outgrow' their symptoms but, unless the immune system is treated, it may be that there is a lull for a short while, before new allergic symptoms emerge, often unconnected by parents with the original allergy.

Causes of Allergies

With allergies in children so much on the increase, it is worth considering the causes, so that parents may help their children to withstand the current trend.

● In the past, babies who were breast-fed for long periods were far less prone to allergies in babyhood or later on than babies fed on cow's milk formulas (see Breast-feeding, page 36). Mother's milk contains important antibodies, known as immunoglobulins, which help to protect the baby's immune system while it is developing, and it also provides vital ingredients for its development, such as gammalinoleic acid (GLA, the now well-known EFA that is found notably in *evening primrose oil*), zinc, selenium, interferon, iron and antioxidants.

● Now, because of a variety of factors, but principally nutritional deficiency and pollution, mother's milk does not protect in the same way, and many breast-fed babies are becoming allergic to substances coming through the breast milk. Drugs and toxins, such as pesticides, herbicides, drug residues in foods, and many other chemicals and heavy metals from the environment in food, water and the air, are taken in through the lungs or the skin and pass through the breast into the baby, where they can interfere with the normal immune function.

● Caffeine, alcohol and nicotine from cigarettes can all play a part.

● It is interesting that vegetarian and vegan mothers have lower levels of hazardous chemicals in their milk compared with meat and fish eaters. Many of these substances – insecticides and dioxin, for instance – collect in fish, eggs and meat.

● Dietary deficiencies of protein, EFAs, vitamins and minerals (notably zinc) can disrupt the formation of prostaglandins and antibodies by the baby's developing immune system.

● However, since the benefits of breast-feeding far outweigh those of bottle feeding, breast-feeding is best for the immune system, especially for the first four to six months of life, until the baby's own system is more mature. Research has shown that breast-feeding at this time boosts immunity and minimizes allergic tendencies and sets the pattern for the future, reducing the likelihood of allergy and auto-immune disease such as diabetes, Crohn's disease and ulcerative colitis in older children and adults.

● Most children with allergies require more EFAs than those without allergies because a major enzyme involved with the metabolism of EFAs is unavailable or does not function as well as it should. The result is that linoleic acid (LA) taken in through the diet is not converted to its usable form, gammalinoleic acid (GLA), and so is not available to the immune system. The tendency to this is inherited from one or other parent, and is most apparent in children with eczema, asthma and hay fever. It is often easily overcome by adding GLA to the diet as well as plenty of foods rich in EFAs.

> ### An Impaired Immune System Can Be Caused By
>
> ☐ Stress
> ☐ Poor diet and nutritional deficiencies
> ☐ Environmental pollution
> ☐ Drugs, including the overuse of antibiotics that can suppress the immune system and upset the intestinal flora, allowing harmful organisms such as *Candida albicans* to flourish
> ☐ Injury or surgery
> ☐ Digestive problems such as poor elimination, candida, enzyme deficiency
> ☐ Inherited susceptibility
> ☐ Genetic problems; damage to chromosome 6, which controls immunity, can cause recurring infections

● If the diet contains plenty of EFAs and GLA and yet allergic symptoms persist, it is likely that there is a deficiency of either vitamins or minerals that are necessary for the enzymes involved with EFA metabolism. This may be caused either by eating depleted foods or foods that rob the body of nutrients or block their availability to the body, or by digestive disorders causing enzyme deficiency or malabsorption, meaning that even if the right foods are eaten, they are not absorbed into the body.

TREATMENT OF THE IMMUNE SYSTEM

Prevention is always better than cure. A wholefood diet, high in organic fruit and vegetables, grains, nuts and seeds, beans and pulses, unrefined oil and oily fish, will lay the foundations for a healthy immune system. Where there is an inherited weakness of the immune system, extra preventative measures may be necessary. These can be used before the onset of symptoms, or, once they have developed, to treat them and prevent the development of chronic problems.

HOW TO BOOST IMMUNITY

Breast Milk Breast-feed your baby for as long as you can. Even if there is no family history of immune problems, it is best to breast-feed exclusively for three to six months and then to introduce new foods slowly, leaving highly allergenic foods, such as wheat, milk, eggs and oranges until last, until the baby is over ten months old, while continuing to breast-feed. If there is a family history of allergy, it would be best to breast-feed almost exclusively for this period of time, during which the mother should avoid excesses of highly allergenic foods, food additives, caffeine, alcohol and cigarettes. Nutritional supplements for either the mother or baby may be necessary should illness or allergy develop. (For more information on breast-feeding see page 36.)

EFAs and GLA Make sure your children get enough EFAs from nuts, seeds, beans and oily fish. Home-grown walnuts, sunflower seeds, haricot and kidney beans are all particularly useful. In addition, give extra oils daily in the form of pure, unrefined **food-grade** linseed oil, or walnut, unhydrogenated sunflower, safflower or soya oil. These oils should all be kept refrigerated so that they do not turn bitter and rancid; if this happens they should not be used. About a tablespoonful of oil needs to be given daily to children; 1 teaspoonful to babies over six months – this can be mixed with fruit juice or made into a dressing using half olive oil, and adding cider vinegar, yoghurt, tahini, honey or herbs to flavour it or to thicken it to resemble mayonnaise. You can also use oils, mixed with butter, as a healthy alternative to hydrogenated margarine. In addition, especially if you have trouble getting your children to take the oil, give it in small amounts through the day, or drop it on to casseroles, soups and stews just before you serve them so that they will not notice.

Evening primrose oil or *blackcurrant seed oil* will provide the body with GLA–EFAs in their usable form. These may be necessary if a child develops allergies or recurrent infections despite the above measures. Start a toddler on one or two 500mg capsules daily. However, doses up to 1 gram (1000mg) may be given to children. *If your child suffers with epilepsy, do not give this before consulting your practitioner.*

Cod Liver Oil Supplements of cod liver oil can also be given, either in capsule form or on the spoon – no more than 1 teaspoonful a day for young children. This may be disguised in the same way as the above oils to make it more palatable. Some flavoured cod liver oils are available on the market. Other fish oil extracts are also available, but these are best taken under professional supervision.

All these oils can also be taken in via the skin. The vegetable and fish oils may not smell very pleasant and could be mixed with a variety of pleasant-smelling essential oils such as *rosewood*, *lavender* or *camomile*. (No more than two drops of essential oil per 5ml of base oil). Rubbing EFAs into the skin is particularly useful for babies – 250mg from a broken capsule can be applied to the inner arm or thigh where it is easily absorbed. You can also use a teaspoon of linseed, walnut, safflower or soya oil to massage the whole body.

Extra Nutrients The nutrients necessary to boost immunity can be increased in the diet of both breast-feeding mothers and children. More magnesium from seafoods, beans and nuts; B vitamins from yeast extract or brewer's yeast; iron from liver, tahini, dried fruits, seeds, pulses, fresh green and yellow vegetables and fruit; zinc from eggs, nuts and seeds, especially pumpkin seeds, oysters and meat; vitamin A from fish and yellow and green vegetables; vitamin C from fresh fruit and vegetables. (For more information on food sources see page 173.)

A diet high in protein will help to build up immunity, while roughage from fruit and vegetables, nuts and seeds, beans and pulses will help to keep the digestive tract working healthily, encourage beneficial gut bacteria to help resist infection, and ensure evacuation of toxins from the system. A diet low in carbohydrates, particularly refined carbohydrates and sugar is recommended. Excess carbohydrates can have a detrimental effect on blood sugar levels and depress immunity.

Cider Vinegar Cider vinegar can be taken in warm water with a teaspoon of honey, which helps to protect against infection in the respiratory and digestive tract.

State of Mind Allergies are closely related to stress, in that a child who is under emotional stress is more likely to develop food and chemical intolerance, as it tends to lower immunity. Negative thoughts and feelings have been shown, through skin tests, to affect local immunity in the skin, while calming thoughts and meditation have been shown to increase the skin's immunity to viruses and the activity of white blood cells in the blood.

Herbs to Boost Immunity

Garlic One clove or two perles morning and night. This is one of nature's best natural antimicrobial products, which can help to prevent bacterial, viral and fungal infections. It has even proved itself effective against infections that have become immune to antibiotics.

Astragalus This famous Chinese herb can be used to increase energy and build resistance to disease.

Chinese Angelica Another famous Chinese herb, Chinese angelica is well known for restoring energy and vitality and enhancing the immune system by its stimulating effect on white blood cell and antibody formation.

Liquorice This can be taken during or after illness to speed recovery and as a tonic during convalescence. It enhances the immune system by stimulating the formation and efficiency of white blood cells and antibodies. It is beneficial to the liver and acts to support the adrenal glands, providing protection from the effects of stress.

Borage The traditional use of borage for depression and stress-related problems suggests a supportive and restorative effect on the adrenal glands. Other hormonal effects include the stimulation of milk production in a breast-feeding mother. It can be used as a tonic for the adrenals, as well as a remedy for fevers and to aid convalescence.

Wild Yam This contains substances related to steroid hormones, which have an anti-inflammatory action, helping to relieve the effects of infection and allergy. It is also a tonic to the liver and digestive tract.

Echinacea One of the best herbal alternatives to antibiotics, echinacea is useful for all chronic and acute bacterial and viral infections. (It needs to be taken every hour or two during acute infections for good effect.) It helps in the cleansing of the blood and lymphatic system and activates white blood cells and antibodies.

Ginseng This remarkable herbal remedy is famous for its ability to boost immunity and energy and to enable the body to cope with stress. *Panax ginseng* (Korean ginseng) is particularly recommended to enhance convalescence for children who are very run down after illness. It is not to be taken during acute illness or if there is inflammation, but it is beneficial for pale, lethargic children, increasing their white blood cell count and helping the liver and spleen in their immunological work.

Myrrh This is a powerful antiseptic, which helps to remove toxins from the stomach and intestines. It should be used only in small amounts.

HOW TO TREAT INFECTIONS

Of all infections, bacterial and viral are the most prevalent, bacteria causing a variety of problems, including throat, ear and chest infections, stomach upsets and some skin problems. Viruses are involved in colds, influenza and infectious diseases such as measles, chicken pox and mumps.

Fasting When a child goes down with any infection the appetite will decrease, so do not give any solid food unless the child is hungry. Fasting helps to boost the immune system. Give plenty of liquid every half hour or so to enhance the elimination of toxins via urine and to prevent dehydration.

Vitamin C Give supplements of vitamin C, 200–500mg three or four times a day to enhance the immune system. If this is more than the body needs it will be excreted via the urine and the worst that will happen will be the onset of diarrhoea. If this occurs, reduce the dose.

Vitamin A Supplements of vitamin A will help the body to resolve infections, particularly viruses, encourage speedy recovery and prevent recurrent infections, particularly among allergic children. Give a dessertspoonful of cod liver oil daily over four or five days (unless the child has diarrhoea), and this will also supply extra EFAs. You can also give carrot juice or carrot soup as part of their liquid intake. Watercress soup not only contains vitamins C and A, but also certain antibiotic substances to help resolve infections.

Garlic Garlic is a wonderful remedy for infections, both viral and bacterial, helping the body to fight off the invaders as it passes through the respiratory, digestive and urinary systems, and throughout the body, reaching even the pores of the skin – as many with a sensitive nose will appreciate. Garlic capsules can be broken open and mixed with a drink or given on a spoon to toddlers, or given as capsules to older children every two or three hours. Garlic honey or juice (see page 109) can also be given. Onions and onion juice are also useful as they, like garlic, contain selenium and other sulphur compounds to ward off infection.

Herbs to Fight Infection Other herbs that will enhance resistance and help fight off infections include *astragalus, camomile, Chinese angelica, cinammon, cleavers, cloves, echinacea, elderflowers, eucalyptus, golden seal, hyssop, liquorice, poke root, red clover, sage, thyme* and *wild indigo.* A choice of these can be taken as warm teas, sweetened with honey if necessary and combined with other herbs more specific to the particular area of the body affected by the infection, and with herbs for fever management (see page 85).

Propolis can be given in honey or a few drops of tincture in a drink. This is an antiseptic material, which bees collect from tree sap to plaster over the hive to keep it clean and protected from infection. Certain substances from propolis, such as flavonoids, help the body to make antibodies and enhance the work of white blood cells in killing harmful bacteria.

ANTIBIOTICS

Antibiotics may be necessary for the treatment of some bacterial infections, notably middle ear infection or streptococcal throat infections, or others that do not respond to other forms of treatment, and they are irrefutably invaluable in some serious acute illness.

To Reduce Antibiotic Side-effects

If your child is prescribed antibiotics, there are several things you can do to prevent side-effects (such as diarrhoea, constipation, abdominal pain) and to support the immune system:

• Give *garlic*, either in perles or honey, to prevent the proliferation of unwanted organisms in the gut, to protect the liver and to boost immunity.

• Give live yoghurt with lactobacillus, or lactobacillus tablets (Acidophilus) to protect the intestinal flora and prevent infection. Lactobacillus produces acids in the gut, and these enhance peristaltic movements and so the elimination of toxins and harmful organisms via the bowel.

• Give cider vinegar and honey and fresh lemon juice to drink to help cleaning of the digestive tact.

• Make sure the child has plenty of liquids to aid elimination of toxins via the kidneys and bowels.

• Make sure the child has plenty of rest to help speed recovery.

• Vitamins can be used, particularly in children who are susceptible to side-effects from antibiotics, notably vitamin C (500mg twice daily) and vitamin E (200iu daily) until the child is quite well again.

• The liver and kidneys are involved with the metabolism and excretion of any drugs in the body and are, therefore, susceptible to stress because of them. Herbs, such as *garlic*, *dandelion root*, *angelica root*, *rosemary* and *Chinese angelica*, support the action of the liver and help it to break down and remove toxins, by stimulating the flow of bile. Herbs, such as *celery seed* and *wild carrot*, as well as B vitamins, magnesium and potassium help to support the kidneys in their eliminative work. Some herbs, such as *dandelion root*, *holy thistle*, *agrimony* and *echinacea*, help the liver repair itself of any damage caused to it by drug therapy.

CANDIDIASIS

If your allergic child does not respond to the avoidance of common allergens in the diet and to the treatment of the immune system through diet and herbs, it may be that candidiasis is the problem. This is particularly prevalent in children who have had frequent infections for which they have been prescribed antibiotics. This yeast-type fungus has an opportunity to flourish when antibiotics disturb the beneficial bacterial population of the gut, which normally keeps such organisms in check. Candida in the gut can cause irritation and inflammation of the gut wall, which may become more permeable and let through potential allergens, such as proteins, as well as intestinal poisons, into the bloodstream. As a result, food allergies may develop, causing a wide variety of allergic responses including eczema, migraine, recurrent infections, recurrent cystitis, skin rashes (including nappy rash), catarrhal congestion, indigestion and wind, bowel problems and depression and lethargy. Candida can also develop in the mouth and vagina, where it is known as thrush.

Candida in the gut can produce toxic substances that are absorbed through the gut wall into the system and that affect the immune and endocrine systems and paralyse T-cells, and it can cause a child to become allergic to intestinal yeasts. Allergies to yeasts and moulds on foods may develop, including allergies to baker's yeast in bread, brewer's yeast and yeast extract, yeasts on fruit (fresh or dried) and fermented products, such as cheese and malt.

POST-VIRAL SYNDROME

The strain that antibiotics (especially when prescribed frequently) impose upon a child's immune system may reduce his or her ability to fight off infection efficiently, thus leading to recurrent infection or post-viral syndrome, in which the child does not recover properly from a simple viral infection for weeks and sometimes months. During this time the child may feel tired and lethargic and suffer symptoms such as bowel disturbances, abdominal pain, wind, nausea, headaches and depression.

Post-viral syndrome is often associated with poor function of the thymus gland, nutritional deficiencies, particularly of vitamin A, B

73

vitamins, magnesium and zinc. It is also linked to food allergies and chronic candidiasis.

Post-viral syndrome is closely related to ME (myalgic encephalomyelitis), a condition of lowered immunity, which is more common in teenagers and adults and which is characterized by tiredness and lethargy, depression, muscle weakness and aching, as well as a wide variety of other symptoms.

Since post-viral syndrome is closely linked to candidiasis, it is worth following a similar line of treatment, as well as general treatment of the immune system (see page 70), using nutrition and herbs.

Treatment of Candidiasis and Post-viral Syndrome

It is certainly worth introducing a yeast-free diet, for in many cases this has a profound effect upon frequent infections and allergies, as well as symptoms of lowered immunity. In addition, give a diet low in sugar (which feeds yeast) and no foods containing yeasts and moulds. **No:**

- ☐ yeasted bread (use soda or unleavened bread instead);
- ☐ cakes and biscuits containing yeast and sugar (use crackers, rice cakes, oatcakes and so on instead);
- ☐ sweets;
- ☐ commercial fruit juices;
- ☐ dried fruits (which contain fruit sugar);
- ☐ vinegar (in salad dressings, mayonnaise, mustard and tomato ketchup, pickles, relishes and so on);
- ☐ cheese;
- ☐ soy sauce;
- ☐ malt (commonly used to flavour breakfast cereals and drinks), brewer's yeast and yeast extract;
- ☐ yeast-containing vitamins;
- ☐ fungi (mushrooms, fungi-containing foods and so on).
- ☐ fresh fruit (which contains fructose) and milk (which contains lactose) should be given in moderation.

Follow the directions for nutrition to boost immunity (see page 70), and give supplements of EFAs, zinc, vitamins A and C and a multi-mineral and vitamin.

- Give *garlic* daily in perles or salads, and lacto-acidophilus in live goat's milk, yoghurt or tablet form.

- Olive oil containing oleic acid is particularly effective in treating candida. You can use this daily in salad dressings, mixed with lemon juice or 2–4 teaspoons (10–20ml) at least dropped on to foods, soups or into drinks through the day.

- Herbs such as *fennel, golden seal, hyssop, marigold, marjoram, rosemary* and *thyme* all have anti-fungal properties and can be infused and taken as teas three times daily, singly or in combination. Flavour with *liquorice*, not honey, if possible.

- Combine these with other herbs to boost the immune system, such as *astralagus, camomile, Chinese angelica, cinnamon, echinacea* and *wild indigo*.

- If there is thrush in the mouth, make a mouth wash from an infusion of *marigold, sage* or *thyme*. Allow it to cool and use one drop of essential oil of either *thyme* or *marjoram* or *oregano* to each cup. Use two or three times daily. Alternatively, use $\frac{1}{4} - \frac{1}{2}$ teaspoon (1–2ml) of tincture of *golden seal, marigold, myrrh* or *sage* diluted in a little water. Lemon juice diluted with equal parts of water is also useful.

HOW TO TREAT ALLERGIES

The cause of an allergic reaction lies not simply in the specific allergen itself, be it grass pollen, the house-dust mite or any other, but rather in all the factors that compromise the efficient functioning of a child's immune system. It is not enough to identify the allergen and remove it, for the malfunctioning immune system remains unchanged, relieved of a burden temporarily, only to turn its attention at a later date to another substance to which the child is frequently exposed. This is confirmed by the fact that many infants who are found to be milk-allergic and are fed on soya products instead, sooner or later begin to react adversely to soya as well. It is the child that needs treatment, not the allergen.

If you can discover which allergens are responsible for sparking off an allergic response, it is certainly worth removing them as far as possible to allow the child some respite while treatment, using nutrition and herbs, is instigated:

• If it is an external or atmospheric allergen, it is often hard to identify the culprit, and even if you do, it can be difficult to remove it from contact with the child – for instance, grass pollen cannot be removed from the atmosphere during the hay fever season. However, if there is a reaction to environmental allergens, there are usually also one or two food substances to which the child reacts, and these are far easier to manipulate once identified.

• If you remove offending foods, the child is able to cope far more effectively with those allergens you are able to do less about. For example, frequently, if you remove wheat (a member of the grass family) from the diet during the hay fever season, the grass pollen is better tolerated by the mucous membranes of the respiratory tract, and hay fever symptoms are dramatically reduced, if not eliminated.

• Similarly, you may find that by removing milk products from the diet, a child who reacts to a beloved pet, be it a cat, a dog or a horse, with rhinitis – sneezing, runny nose and eyes and often wheezing – may be able to show affection to the pet without suffering the consequences.

How to Identify Allergens and Remove Them from the Diet

Many foods – milk produce, wheat, eggs and sugar are eaten every day, perhaps twice or three times a day, from infancy through to old age. These constitute the most common allergens, perhaps because we are over-exposed to them or because they have been produced with the use of chemicals or because, in the case of sugar, they depress the immune system.

Most Common Dietary Allergens When a baby first takes solid foods there may be a reaction such as irritability, restlessness, colic, catarrh, respiratory infections or eczema. This is frequently not recognized as a food reaction, and the baby continues to be given it and some minor symptoms persist. Some time later, more allergic symptoms develop. If the culprit food is omitted from the diet, these can clear

within three days to three weeks, but, in some children this can take longer. There may be withdrawal symptoms, which can present as a worsening of the problem before it gets better. If the food is given in the next few weeks, a strong reaction may develop over the next day or two, either the same as the original symptoms or slightly different.

The foods and substances most likely to cause allergic reactions are:
- ☐ Wheat
- ☐ Milk produce (and sometimes beef)
- ☐ Eggs (and sometimes chicken)
- ☐ Oranges (and often other citrus fruits)
- ☐ Potatoes, tomatoes (also, often peppers and aubergines, which are in the same family)
- ☐ Maize
- ☐ Gluten (protein found in oats, wheat, barley and rye)
- ☐ Food additives
- ☐ Agricultural chemicals (such as pesticides and herbicides in foods)
- ☐ Fungi and yeasts on foods (on grains, for example)
- ☐ Chocolate, tea and coffee
- ☐ Cane and beet sugar
- ☐ Pork
- ☐ Peanuts

The longer an offending food is removed from the diet, the better a child is able to tolerate it later. It is best to avoid the food for at least two months, after which it may be gradually reintroduced, in small amounts initially, once every five days. If no symptoms develop, introduce it more frequently, every four days, then three, then two and so on and in larger amounts. If symptoms develop, withdraw the food completely until they clear, and then re-introduce it more gradually. You may find that for several months your child can tolerate the offending food in small amounts only, every four or five days. The child should be treated until the food can be tolerated in moderate amounts on a regular basis. This may take months and sometimes even years. Some food allergies are called 'fixed' because they tend to last for life – for example, those to shellfish, strawberries and penicillin.

It may not be clear which food or foods your child is reacting to, as many food allergies are 'masked' and do not necessarily erupt each time the child eats the offending food. The best

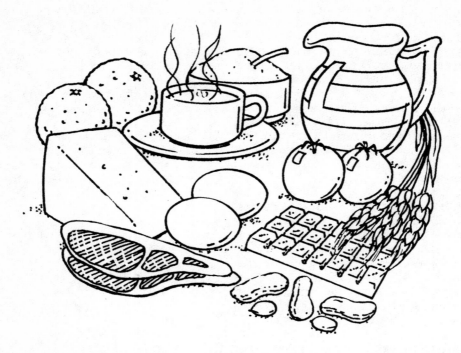

thing is to examine the child's diet for common allergens that crop up frequently and especially those that the child loves or craves, and remove them – for, cruelly, it is usually those that are responsible. Often when you remove foods that a child craves, withdrawal symptoms may present as malaise and a variety of other symptoms, which disappear when the food is given again. Do not be fooled into thinking that, because the child feels better, that food is good for them. It is probably the culprit and not the cure!

Remove one food that crops up repeatedly or the child craves, at a time or choose a common allergen, such as wheat or milk, and do not reintroduce it for at least a month, during which time you can assess any improvement in the symptoms. If there is none, try the next suspected food for the same length of time. If the symptoms are better, continue to avoid the food while the child is treated. Alternatively, you can omit a few suspected foods simultaneously, which may be difficult practically, but may well be worthwhile if your child is reacting to several different foods at the same time.

If you have removed a few possible allergens and there is no positive response, it may be that the child's immune system is too overburdened by environmental stresses to improve without further treatment, or that there are serious nutritional deficiencies. If so, treatment needs to involve not only environmental measures and avoidance of as many pollutants as possible, but also nutritional treatment to right deficiencies and to help the body to eliminate its toxic overload.

If you decide to try eliminating foods from your child's diet for more than a few weeks, this is best done with the advice of a professional herbalist or allergy specialist, otherwise you may be compromising the child's nutrition.

The elimination of foods from the diet can be difficult socially for you and the child, especially in the first month while you are waiting to see if symptoms improve. Once you have determined which foods are the offenders, you have to make a choice: do you allow the child the odd indiscretion, knowing what it may lead to, or do you keep strictly to the diet? You may, however, find that the child can tolerate the offending food occasionally, and gradually more so as he or she improves.

Whether or not you can identify the allergen, you can treat the child, although clear results may emerge more rapidly when offending allergens are removed. The child needs to be treated as a whole, paying attention to possible causes of the allergy (see page 67), including emotional problems and stress, poor diet, and an unhealthy lifestyle (not enough sleep, relaxation, fresh air and exercise and over-exposure to harmful chemicals and so on), as well as specific physical weaknesses or imbalances, such as a weak digestion or an inherited tendency. This may prove a complex process, and you may need to consult your local herbal practitioner for further advice and discussion.

Through the right treatment, the general health and vitality of the child will improve, making him or her better able to withstand exposure to the allergens, at least in moderate amounts, which will mean that you can then start to re-introduce offending foods gradually.

• Follow recommendations for boosting the immune system using nutrition and herbs (see page 70).

• Emotional difficulties, stresses at home or at school should be taken into consideration, and as much support provided as possible (see Nervous System, page 122).

• The proper function of the digestive tract and the liver are vital to the prevention and treatment of the problems of the immune system (see also Digestive System, page 129). Disruption of the gut bacteria can cause abnormal bowel overgrowth and candidiasis (page 73), which can lead to digestive disturbances, such as chronic constipation and diarrhoea, and result in absorption of toxins into the system, which further compromise the immune system. The irritation and inflammation thereby created in the wall of the gut can make it more permeable to toxins from the intestines as well as whole proteins from foods, predisposing the child to food allergies.

• Allergies to food can be related not only to disturbances in gut flora but also to deficiency or disruption of digestive enzymes. Stress has a well-documented effect on the function of the digestive tract (see Nervous System, page 122) and could account for enzyme deficiency.

Dietary Advice for Allergies

• It is worth starting each meal with raw foods, for these, especially salads, stimulate the secretion of digestive enzymes and help the digestive system to break down foods efficiently. This makes it less likely that large, undigested molecules, especially whole proteins, will pass through the gut walls, to be misinterpreted as alien substances by the immune system, which would then rally its defences unnecessarily to create an allergic response.

• Tea drinking, especially without milk, inhibits the secretion of digestive enzymes and can, therefore, predispose to food allergies.

• Herbs, such as *borage, camomile, cinnamon, echinacea, lemon balm, liquorice, red clover, sage, wild yam* and *yarrow* can be given singly or in combination to enhance the function of the immune system and to help build resistance to allergies. They may have to be taken over several months for good effect.

• In addition, *camomile* and *yarrow* should be given daily as a tea to any allergic child. They soothe the allergic response and inhibit the production of histamine, which is responsible for many of the inflammatory symptoms involved.

• *Nettles* in tea, soups or stews also have a good reputation for calming the allergic response.

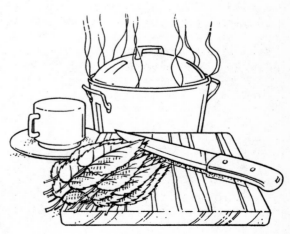

- Essential oils of *camomile, lemon balm* and *yarrow* can be used in a variety of ways – in the bath, as inhalations and for massage.

- Vitamin C supplements (500mg twice daily) and magnesium tablets (500mg daily) are natural antihistamines and should be administered daily until the allergic symptoms subside. Giving 1 teaspoon of sodium bicarbonate (baking soda) dissolved in a little water can reduce acute symptoms and can be given every few hours when necessary. (See also specific allergies in ailments section.)

Environmental Control for Allergies

Even though it is easier to work with and manipulate the dietary intake of a child rather than the environment, it is still worth thinking about what changes can be made to reduce the potential allergens around an allergic child.

- Maintaining adequate humidity in the house atmosphere is important, especially if there is central heating. Keep windows open, even in the winter where possible, and put saucers of water by fires or radiators. Showers and baths, drying clothes on radiators and tumble driers will all release moisture into the atmosphere. Humidifiers can be easily installed or portable ones can be carried from room to room; these are particularly useful at night in the bedroom of a child with an allergy or respiratory infection.

- Because dust, harbouring the house-dust mite and infection, is a common allergen, it is important to keep it to a minimum and to prevent disturbing it too vigorously when cleaning so that it blows into the atmosphere and simply lands elsewhere. Use a vacuum cleaner rather than a broom or duster, keep surfaces free of too many objects that collect dust and keep those that need to be stood on shelves, such as books and toys, in closed cupboards if possible. The house-dust mite tends to live in mattresses, so these should be cleaned regularly or covered with a special fabric to reduce allergic symptoms.

- Avoid the use of wool and synthetic fibres in clothes next to an allergic child's skin, and be careful not to let a child who is sensitive to wool play on an all-wool carpet. Cotton underclothes are the least irritating and also let the skin breathe properly in a way that synthetic fibres may not. Quilts or duvets on beds may be helpful alternatives to the woollen blankets in a wool-sensitive child, but some children may be sensitive to down and feathers.

- Pay attention to the chemicals and pollutants you have in the house, whether these are from cigarette smoke, furniture polish, or bleach in the sink and biological washing powders. These environmental pollutants can be avoided or exchanged for more environmentally friendly products that, in many cases, can be very helpful with regard to relieving allergic symptoms. Smoky fires, faulty heaters and cigarettes all give out carbon monoxide, which is linked with an increased incidence of respiratory infections and allergy.

- Tap water can cause a number of problems. It may be contaminated with agricultural chemicals, nitrates, lead, aluminium, chlorine and fluoride, all of which can be implicated in allergies. Allowing the tap to run for a few minutes before using it will reduce the concentration of harmful substances, some of which can also be reduced by the use of water filters.

CHAPTER 8

HOME NURSING

The home and family environment represent the most important factors influencing a child's health. Parents provide their children with the raw ingredients for their developing health – good food, healthy lifestyle, fresh air, warmth and hygiene, as well as love and support.

In almost every case, illness starts in the home. By their intimate knowledge of their child, the parents will be aware of subtle changes in the child's appearance and behaviour and other nuances in the pattern of the child's health, which may indicate the onset of illness. They have the opportunity to introduce therapeutic measures, with diet and herbs, the minute they sense some imbalance, which is far more valuable than waiting until frank symptoms manifest themselves, and then rushing the child to the doctor when the illness has got out of hand.

Even though most parents may rely considerably on the judgement and responsibility of their family practitioner, it is actually the family who are in the best position to determine how the symptoms are progressing, whether the child is ill or just off colour, whether he or she is upset physically or emotionally, whether it really is 'tummy ache' or the child does not want to go to school, or whether it is a cry for love and attention. Over time parents develop their own instinctive nursing skills and means of interpreting symptoms, and they have a sense of when symptoms are mild or serious, based on their observation of the child and their own emotional response to him or her. This is not to be disregarded, either by parents who lack confidence in their own abilities or by the practitioner who, although having a greater medical knowledge, has less understanding of the individual child concerned.

Most common ailments may, in fact, be dealt with perfectly adequately at home and do not require intervention by the doctor. Most childhood illnesses are mild and self-limiting, and generally, if left to their own devices, the child's healing energies will quickly have the child up and about in no time. This process may well be enhanced by the use of various natural remedies, rather than over-the-counter medicines – for coughs and colds for example. In most cases it is generally a matter of caring for the child, giving plenty of love and reassurance, and combining rest with some home treatments and basic nursing skills.

In the days of the extended family, nursing skills were more extensive and comprehensive. Knowledge was handed down from one generation to another. Now, when the comparatively isolated nuclear family is more usual, these basic skills can often be sorely lacking, and the responsibility for a family's health has largely shifted over to the overworked family doctor.

Without the support, reassurance and knowledge within the extended family, it is easy for a mother on her own at home with a sick child to lose confidence and panic or simply feel out of her depth. Most parents are reluctant to bother their doctors about minor symptoms they feel they should be able to cope with at home, but the problem is being able to differentiate with confidence between minor and serious symptoms, and at what point it is necessary to call in professional help. A child's metabolism works more quickly than an adult's. Their breathing is faster, their heartbeat is more rapid, and they consume proportionately more food and drink than adults. They also become ill more rapidly, which can be worrying for the parents until they accept this as normal, and happily they also recover more quickly than adults. In health, children have far greater vital energy than most adults, which makes them very resilient on the whole and able to bounce back to life with a speedy recovery.

In the modern nuclear family it is important for every parent to acquire a basic knowledge of home nursing skills and home treatments, and to learn to recognize the difference between minor illnesses and those that are more serious, as well as to trust their own judgement a little more. It is hoped that this manual will go some way towards teaching these skills, to be used in conjunction with the advice of your local herbal practitioner and doctor.

CHILDHOOD ILLNESS

While a child's vital force works to maintain homoeostasis and health, if too many pathogenic influences – poor diet, lack of fresh air, a new or virulent infection, for instance – overburden it, then 'sickness' results. Unwanted organisms and toxins, which are usually dealt with by the body's immune and eliminative system, begin to accumulate in the body. However, the healing energy of the body rallies its defences and directs its force towards throwing them off. To do this, energy is withdrawn from normal daily processes, such as digestion and assimilation, and directed towards cleansing and eliminating the waste products through the natural channels – bowels, kidneys, skin and lungs – and the stimulation of the immune system. The various signs, symptoms, 'illnesses' and conditions are not so much signs of disease as evidence of the body carrying out its own self-cleansing process.

We can enhance the speed of this healing process by avoiding overburdening our children's bodies with heavy food while the digestive energy is involved elsewhere and refraining from giving 'remedies' to suppress the action of the vital force. It is inadvisable to give medicines indiscriminately to stop vomiting or diarrhoea, or to bring down a mild fever, as these are the very mechanisms we have for warding off disease as quickly as possible. Such symptoms could be interpreted as signs of *health* not disease. Each case has to be judged on its own merits, for obviously if either vomiting or diarrhoea persist too long or the fever is rising quickly, some treatment may be required. However, suppression of the efforts of the vital force will only serve to push the illness further into the body or into a more chronic state. As the defensive system is weakened by such suppression, it is less able to ward off subsequent threats to health and this predisposes to further illness.

There are, for example, many babies and children who suffer from frequent colds, coughs, catarrh and ear infections. The mucus produced in the nose, throat or chest results from irritation of their sensitive linings (mucous membranes) from infection, environmental chemicals, or internal or external allergens. The excess mucus acts protectively to dilute the irritants and minimize the damage to the mucous membranes. Anti-catarrhal medicines or astringent nose drops are directly antagonistic to the inherent healing action of the body, as antibiotics are to the function of the immune system, and its strength is thereby depleted, its efforts reduced and only a half-hearted attempt at elimination of the irritants is possible. The outcome of this is the development of chronic catarrh and/or frequent respiratory infections. As simple symptoms are suppressed and illness is pushed further into the body, and as our healing energy is depleted, so the nature of the subsequent illness is changed, very often to that of a more serious nature. A case of infantile eczema may be 'cured' by hydrocortisone cream (a steroid cream), but asthma may well develop later as a result.

ANTIBIOTICS – THE ABUSED 'WONDER DRUGS'

Antibiotics are a wonderful invention for acute, serious infection. They have saved lives, but may not be necessary for mild, self-limiting acute infections. Far better to reserve them for stubborn infections that respond to nothing else or for rapidly escalating symptoms, when time is of the essence. They are often prescribed more to calm the mother than for the health of the infant or child, or for minor infections, or even for an infection that could be viral and so not responsive to antibiotics. They are often given before a proper diagnosis is established: 'Try these and if there is no change come back for further tests.' It is estimated that between 75 and 90 per cent of childhood respiratory infections are related to viruses that do not respond to antibiotics, and yet antibiotics are prescribed in over 75 per cent of all childhood illness.[1] Since infection is generally accompanied by fever, which in itself enhances the resolution of infection, whether viral or bacterial, it is clearly illogical to suppress fever with antipyretic (fever-reducing) drugs while, at the same time, administering antibiotics. Many people are now aware of the side-effects of antibiotics. The main one is the disturbance of the beneficial bacteria that live in the body. These bacteria, comprising about five hundred species, live in the intestines and are vital for normal digestion, metabolism, synthesis of vitamins and elimination of toxins. Their destruction allows the hostile forms of bacteria and fungus (such as *Candida albicans*), which they normally keep in check, to proliferate. This can lead to digestive problems, loss of nutrients, disturbed bowel action, tiredness, malaise, headache, insomnia and lowered resistance, predisposing to further infections, which can be resistant to the first antibiotic. This warrants the use of more powerful antibiotics, and so the cycle continues. A study published in the *Lancet* in 1975 found that infection was three times more frequent in those undergoing surgery who had received routine antibiotics than those who had not.[2]

Other side-effects of antibiotics include allergies. These can result when yeasts and harmful bacteria damage the intestinal walls, which allows seepage of intestinal poisons. Research has shown that this may be linked to food allergies and eczema.[3]

The obvious answer to avoiding the use of antibiotics is preventative medicine; parents can use diet and herbs to boost their children's immunity on a daily basis and incorporate them simply and effortlessly into everyday life. If a certain pattern of health begins to develop in a child with a particular susceptibility to certain symptoms, it is far better to look for causes than constantly to seek to eliminate the symptoms as quickly as possible.

There are myriad books on herbs for a whole host of symptoms and diseases, but it is still very easy to feel quite at sea amid a confusion of information, when acute illness arises and you need to act quickly. For advice and support, therefore, it is worth paying a visit to your local consultant herbalist so that, having established a relationship, you can call on his or her help at short notice when necessary. Naturally, many parents will not want to rely over-much on home diagnosis and nursing skills, and a visit to or from the herbalist may well provide the necessary confidence and reassurance that will go hand-in-hand with the use of a manual of this kind.

FIRST SIGNS OF ILLNESS

The first signs of imbalance or illness vary from one child to another and will differ from one age group to another. The one constant is that there will be a departure from the child's *normal* behaviour, routine and appearance. Is your child who usually has a large appetite

suddenly off his food? While it is normal for a baby to sleep on and off through the day, it is not normal for a six-year-old to do the same.

Furthermore, when your child is ill, you need to be able to detect the subtle differences between what is *normal* for that particular illness and what is not. For example, if a child has mumps it is normal for the temperature to rise and the salivary glands in front of and beneath the ears and chin to swell up, causing pain on swallowing and a dry mouth. Mumps is normally a mild disease. However, if after ten days the child is still unwell and develops a severe headache and a stiff neck, it could mean that mumps has developed into encephalitis or meningitis and the doctor must be called immediately.

If you feel that your child is off-colour or unwell, but he or she is too young to tell you what is wrong, there are several questions you can ask yourself. Is the child:

☐ Off his or her food?
☐ Less active than usual? Tired and lethargic? More restless than usual?
☐ Behaving differently? Crying more, or bad tempered? Withdrawn?
☐ Having disturbed nights or wanting to sleep more in the daytime?

The above are all quite normal in most minor and self-limiting illnesses.

When to Call in Professional Help

☐ Persistent fever of 102°F (39°C)
☐ Raised temperature and a history of convulsions
☐ Raised temperature and convulsions
☐ A temperature that drops and rises again suddenly
☐ A temperature below 95°F (35°C) accompanied by cold skin, drowsiness, quietness and listlessness
☐ Diarrhoea and/or vomiting for more than 6 hours in a baby
☐ Prolonged and violent vomiting
☐ Nausea, vomiting or diarrhoea with abdominal pains and fever
☐ A baby is off its food for more than a day or two and does not seem to be thriving
☐ Laboured breathing, with ribs sharply drawn in with each breath. (Bear in mind

that the breathing rate varies according to the age of the child. A new-born baby breathes 50 times a minute, a six-year-old 30 times, and a ten-year-old 25 times a minute.[4])

☐ A rash; all rashes require attention, for proper diagnosis, as they could indicate notifiable childhood infection such as measles

Emergency Signs: Call Doctor Immediately

☐ The child has profuse vomiting or diarrhoea or has not passed water for 24 hours
☐ The eyes are dull, glazed or sunken
☐ The soft spot on the baby's head bulges or sinks in
☐ The breathing alters and becomes shallow or rapid, or the skin turns pale or blue
☐ The child's consciousness changes — drowsy from dehydration; slipping between near unconsciousness and being alert; disoriented
☐ The child has nausea, dizziness, headache, drowsiness or blurred vision after a recent fall or blow to the head
☐ The child has a convulsion
☐ There is a sharp pain in the right abdomen with nausea

Other medical emergencies for which you should seek immediate professional assistance are:

☐ Choking that cannot be cleared immediately
☐ Heavy bleeding from a wound for more than a few minutes
☐ Bad burn
☐ Chemicals in eyes or mouth
☐ Animal or snake bite
☐ Suspected broken bones

FEVER

Fever is a natural accompaniment to many infections. The popular response to a child's fever is an attempt to suppress it immediately. However, this may not actually be best for the child.

Fever is a symptom of the body's fight against the illness. It is not a disease and it may well be a friend. An infection begins when certain micro-organisms have a chance to multiply in the body. As viruses and bacteria are broken down by the cells of the immune system, toxic breakdown products called pyrogens are released. Pyrogens raise the setting of the body's internal thermostat. As a result, the metabolism of the body is increased and this enables the infecting organisms to be combated quickly and efficiently. In fact, fever itself has an antibiotic and antiviral effect. For example, interferon, which is released during a viral infection, is more effective when the child has fever than when the temperature remains normal. When the fever is no longer required by the body and the infection is successfully resolved, the thermostat will reset itself.

Fevers produced by childhood illness are regarded by herbalists as a strong and vital response to the accumulation of toxins in the body. These toxins are derived from a variety of sources: pollution in the atmosphere, chemicals in food, water, poor nutrition, sluggish elimination of waste products, too little fresh air and exercise, to name but a few.

It is interesting to consider at this point why some children develop an infection while others living or playing close to them do not. While bacteria and viruses have taken the blame for the onset of infection, in actual fact they are perceived by the herbalist as merely precipitating factors in disease, not the real underlying cause. The predisposing factor that allows the bacteria or virus to proliferate in the body is a state of lowered resistance or vitality related to an accumulation of toxins in the system. What is of most significance, therefore, is the patient, not the disease. Herbal treatment is aimed towards the individual concerned and his or her particular pattern of health. It is significant that the herbs that would be used to help resolve the infection not only encourage elimination of waste materials and toxins but also provide the weakened system with vitamins, minerals and trace elements to boost general health. In this sense, the idea of a herbal tonic comes into its own.

Children growing up in the 1990s may well need periodic times of cleansing the system, and a mild fever is a good way to do it. This provides an opportunity to give the child's system a rest from solid food and the accumu-

Fever	Possible Illness	Fever	Possible Illness
Fever + runny nose, sneezing, cough	probably a common cold	Fever + runny nose, sore red eyes, red spots, malaise	measles
Fever + sore throat, pain on swallowing, malaise	tonsilitis or viral throat infection	Fever + itchy red spots, which quickly turn into blisters, starting on the body	chicken pox
Fever + hoarseness	laryngitis	Fever + sore throat and a rash of pinhead-size red dots like a scarlet flush and red bumps on tongue	scarlet fever
Fever + swollen neck glands, sore throat, tiredness and malaise	glandular fever		
Fever + aches and pains, malaise, sore throat, cough, runny nose	influenza	Fever + swollen face and chin, difficulty swallowing	mumps
Fever + runny or blocked nose, earache, or if young crying and pulling on one ear	middle ear infection (*otitis media*)	Fever + frequency and soreness/ burning passing water	urinary tract infection
Fever + catarrh, cough	bronchitis	Fever + diarrhoea, vomiting, nausea	gastric flu or gastro-enteritis or food poisoning
Fever + catarrh, rapid or difficult breathing or bad colour	bronchiolitis or pneumonia – **consult your doctor immediately**	Fever + stiff neck, headache, avoidance of bright light	possible meningitis – **consult your doctor immediately**

lation of more waste matter for a few days, and allows the eliminative pathways a chance to throw off toxins through the increase in metabolism experienced with a fever. Sweating, a vital pathway of elimination, can be encouraged by the use of herbal teas. Drinking plenty of liquids can not only encourage sweating but also elimination through the kidneys and bladder. Herbs with mild laxative properties may also be helpful in some instances to speed the process.

As long as the child is basically healthy and robust, most minor diseases accompanied by a fever will be easily overcome, and the child will be healthier as a result of this cleansing process. Some believe that, if properly treated, fevers provide the opportunity not only to throw off toxins accumulated during the child's life but also perhaps toxins inherited from the parents at the embryonic stage of development. It is easy to see, therefore, how unwise standard suppression of fever may be. So rather than the popular perception of illness and fever as something to be eliminated at all costs, perhaps we can take a new look at this concept and see it as a positive protection from serious illness rather than exposing us to it.

A child's general health is going to determine to a large extent his or her reaction to bacterial or viral illness and fever. A well-nourished child, fed on wholefoods and plenty of fresh fruit and vegetables rather than on refined carbohydrates and sugar, should produce a healthy response, with a moderate fever, good sweating and good rash in the eruptive diseases such as chicken pox and measles. The illness should be resolved quickly in this way. It is a more healthy response than a mild fever, light sweating, little rash and malaise that may persist for weeks.

Most childhood infections that are accompanied by fever require the same basic treatment, whether it is a cold, mumps, measles, tonsilitis, laryngitis or gastric 'flu. This consists of a combination of fever management (see page 85), plenty of rest, frequent liquid intake and a short fast with the use of natural remedies to facilitate the process and the child's recovery, from the 'herbal medicine chest' – antiseptics, febrifuges, laxatives and cleansing herbs, and vegetable and fruit juices.

Taking a Child's Temperature

It is important to bear in mind that the body's temperature has normal variations depending on the level of activity, the ambient temperature and the time of day.

Rectal temperatures are normally 0.6°F higher than oral temperatures, and oral temperatures are about 1°F higher than armpit temperatures. Always use the same location when checking the temperature regularly to avoid confusion. Also, use the same thermometer as readings may vary slightly.

Rectal Readings With small children it may well be best to take a rectal reading, for it is more reliable. They cannot keep a thermometer under the tongue, and an armpit reading may not be very accurate. Use a special rectal thermometer, which is shorter and has a rounder end than an oral one. Wipe clean with alcohol after use. If you have a baby or toddler, the easiest way to do this is to take the child on your lap, lying on his or her tummy with the bottom up (see illustration above). Place the heel of your hand firmly on the small of the back and make sure the child's knees are not underneath so that he or she can get up. Open the buttocks with your thumb and index finger of the same hand, and insert the lubricated end of the thermometer with the other, a third to a half the way in (only 1in (2.5cm) in babies). You can read the temperature while it is still

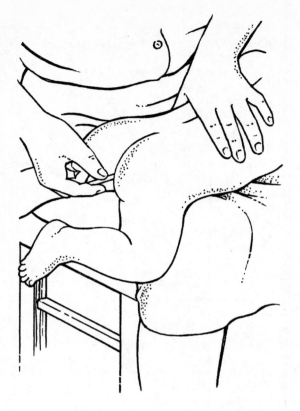

there. It will rise rapidly and then stop, at which point you can take the thermometer out.

Use of Indicator Strips Indicator strips can also be used for babies and young children but depend on the child keeping still for one minute while the strip is pressed against the forehead. The body heat causes chemicals in the strip to change colour, which gives an indication of the approximate temperature. It is not a very accurate way to assess temperature but may well be useful if a child objects to taking the temperature elsewhere.

Normal body temperature is 96.8–98.6°F (36–37°C). A fever is said to exist if a temperature is over approximately 100°F (37.8°C). If you have a baby whose temperature remains above this despite tepid sponging, or a child with a persistent fever of over 103°F consult your doctor.

Of most concern when a baby or child has a persistently raised temperature is the possibility of convulsion (see page 157). Although most children are unlikely to experience convulsions, even with a high fever, some children have a tendency to them. The younger the child and the higher the fever, the more likely a convulsion; hence the need for tepid sponging during fever, especially in a baby. Convulsions tend to be preceded by fever associated with irritability and trembling. *Roseola infantum* is an unusual viral infection causing a red rash of spots and high fever, which is more commonly associated with convulsions than other infectious diseases.

Treating a Fever

General Treatment of Fevers

If your child has a fever, make sure he or she drinks plenty of fluids and only eats lightly. Liquid is essential to encourage sweating, to cool the body and to prevent dehydration.

• Dress the child lightly and put to bed.

• Keep the room at a temperature that is comfortable and the bed out of the sun. If the fever is no higher than 101–102°F (38.3–38.8°C) leave the body to its own devices.

• If it is higher, it can cause the child to feel uncomfortable and often quite unwell and could, if left, lead to dehydration. Take the clothes off and sponge your child down with tepid water. Do not dry the skin afterwards as natural evaporation of the water has cooling effects. Do not stop until the fever is reduced to 102°F (38.8°C), even if the child shivers or has goose pimples, but do not persist for longer than half an hour or more frequently than every two hours. Then cover the naked child with a sheet, check the temperature every 20–30 minutes, and administer drinks as often as possible to replace fluid loss through increased sweating.

• Give supplements of vitamin C, 200–500mg three or four times a day to enhance the immune system. If this is more than the body needs it will be excreted via the urine, and the worst that will happen will be the onset of diarrhoea. If this occurs, reduce the dose.

Herbal Treatment of Fevers

• **Herbal teas** can be employed in a variety of different ways. They can be taken as hot or warm drinks as frequently as possible, they can be used for tepid sponging, or poured into the bath water for the child. They can also be used as hand and foot baths.

The following herbs can be used to encourage sweating and thereby reduce fever, while at the same time they encourage the body's fight against the infection (see Immune System, page 71): Use two teaspoons of dried herb to each ½ pint (300ml) of boiling water or prepare as a standard infusion (see page 23). Choose from the following which can be used either singly or in mixtures to taste: *basil, boneset, borage, camomile, catnip, cinnamon, echinacea, elderflower, ginger, ground ivy, hyssop, lavender, lemon balm, limeflowers, meadowsweet, peppermint, red clover, rosemary, self heal, vervain, violet flowers* and *yarrow*. Add honey, or dilute with water to taste. The important thing is to get your child to drink the tea, either by the cupful every hour or two, or otherwise in smaller amounts every 15–30 minutes. You can alternate them with fruit juices or water. You can also ring the changes and try different mixtures to find the most acceptable to your child.

• **Camomile tea** is a favourite remedy to many, known through the Beatrix Potter stories, for Peter Rabbit was in the habit of taking camomile when he felt unwell. Not only does it enhance the immune response and reduce fever, but it also relaxes baby or child suffi-

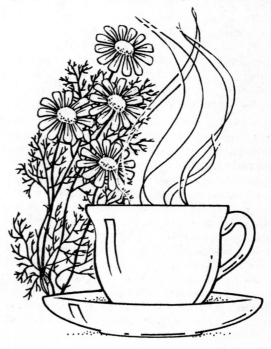

ciently to ensure a good sleep. Rest is probably the single most beneficial factor in speeding recovery in babies and children. It allows the vital force to direct all its healing energy to the problem in hand. *Lavender, lemon balm* and *limeflowers* work similarly. They are all pleasant tasting and can be taken copiously. Sweeten with honey if required.

• **A combined tea of elderflower, peppermint and yarrow** is a famous old recipe for feverish states to encourage sweating.

Cinnamon and Ginger Tea

This delicious tea is simple to make.

1 tablespoon of fresh grated ginger
1 teaspoon cinnamon powder (broken sticks)
1 teaspoon broken licorice sticks

Bring to the boil in 2 pints of water, cover and simmer for 10 minutes. Children over two may have, on average, 1 cupful every two hours sweetened with honey if required. Dilute with half water for 1–2 year olds.

• **Garlic** is renowned for helping the fight against infection and also for encouraging sweating. An older child may even enjoy some chopped raw garlic in a spoonful of honey or in a little milk. If not, and for younger children, three garlic perles can be given a day with a drink. Garlic is one of the most effective antimicrobial herbs, acting on bacteria, viruses and parasites in the gut. It can be used for all infectious conditions, whether of the respiratory, digestive or urinary systems.

• **Limeflowers, camomile** and **elderflowers** are considered to be some of the best diaphoretics, especially for use with children. Two paediatricians at Chicago University, Traismann and Hardy, ran some very interesting trials using limeflowers. Fifty-five children with influenza symptoms were treated with limeflowers, and bed-rest, and at most one or two aspirin tablets; thirty-seven other children were given the above, as well as sulphonamides; and sixty-seven other children were only given antibiotics. Those given only limeflowers and bed-rest recovered most quickly and developed the least complications such as

middle ear infection. The children given sulphonamides and antibiotics took longer to recover and developed more complications. The researchers came out ten to one in favour of limeflower tea.[5] They recommended that trivial childhood illness should not be treated with such drugs, except when complications develop, in which case they may be more applicable.

Limeflower, elderflower and camomile tea should be taken as hot as possible for best sudorific effects (to enhance sweating). Two or three teaspoons of equal parts of these herbs can be used to $\frac{1}{2}$ pint (300ml) of boiling water, infused for 5–10 minutes and taken immediately several times a day.

• **Wormwood** (*Artemisia absinthium*), a very bitter herb and a beautiful shrub that grows easily in temperate climates, has a strengthening effect when used in infectious diseases, particularly for colds and influenza.[6] You may add a few leaves, fresh from the garden, or dried, to other herbal teas given, which may disguise the bitter taste, or chop the leaves finely and take them in a teaspoonful of honey. You could also use a strong wormwood tea as a disinfectant spray for the room, or to sponge or bathe the child.

• **Echinacea** (*Echinacea purpura* and *E. angustifolia*) is one of the most famous remedies to enhance resistance (see Immune System, page 71) in all kinds of infectious diseases, particularly colds and influenza. It should be taken as soon as the first symptoms appear, every two to three hours for the first two days. It is a member of the daisy family and makes a pretty garden plant. All parts of the plant are used. This too can be added to other more pleasant-tasting herbs such as *mint* and *lemon balm*.

• **Hemp agrimony** (*Eupatorium cannabinum*) is another member of the daisy family that grows in profusion in temperate climates. The whole part of the plant can be used to enhance resistance to infection. Like *echinacea*, its main use is in combating viral infection, particularly influenza-like conditions.

• **Meadowsweet** is known as the herbal aspirin and can be taken in any instance where aspirin would be used, but without the side-effects:

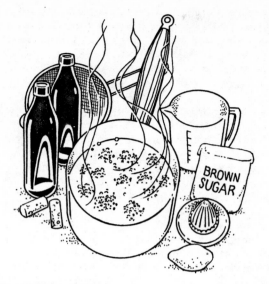

Meadowsweet Syrup

Put 20 flowering heads of meadowsweet, removed from stems, in a saucepan and cover them with cold water. Bring to the boil, cover and simmer for 10 minutes. Strain. Add 4 tablespoons of lemon juice. Measure the liquid. For each 1½ pints (900ml) of liquid add 1lb (500g) of preferably raw sugar. Heat gradually until the sugar has dissolved. Boil for 5 minutes. Skim. Leave to cool. Store in dark bottles with screw-on caps or corks.

This can be diluted with water or soda and taken two or three times a day, it makes a very pleasant drink, or a juice to add to fresh fruit salad or ice-cream.

Beetroot in Treatment of Fevers

The red pigment, betanin, in beetroot (*Beta vulgaris*) has been found to have the effect of enhancing the immune system. During a fever, when fasting, it can be taken as juice (do not be concerned if urine or stool turn red – this is quite normal).

Essential Oils in Treatment of Fevers

Essential oils can also be used effectively to treat fevers. Add a few drops to tepid water to sponge the body down, or to a lukewarm bath to bathe in, or for hand and foot baths, repeated frequently. You can wring a cloth out in cold water with a few drops of *mint oil* and apply frequently to the head, especially if the fever is accompanied by headache. *Lavender* and *camo-*

mile oil will both help to reduce fever as well as relax the child enough to ensure rest for recovery. *Eucalyptus oil* can be used as a disinfectant. Add a few drops to water in a plant spray, and spray around the room at frequent intervals. *Lavender* and *rosemary oil* can be used in the same way.

Diet during a Fever

'Feed a cold and starve a fever' is a maxim you must have heard many times. Does it mean that one should feed a child who has a cold, but starve one with a fever? Or that *if* you feed a cold you will then have to starve a fever? Either way it confirms that the best way to treat a fever is through fasting. Most babies and children have a natural inclination not to eat until they feel better. Over-concern to keep your child's strength up, may lead you to overburden your child with food at a time when he or she has little spare energy for digestion during the recovery process. Remember that it may diminish the force of this healing process and slow recovery down or predispose to complications.

Preferably, little or no food should be given to the child during the fever or while there is no appetite. Plain water with fresh lemon squeezed into it can be given frequently; it is refreshing and cooling as well as antiseptic. Once the fever has abated, the child feels better and the appetite is returning, fruit juices can be given initially. The best juices at this stage include blackberry, gooseberry, lemon juice with honey, mulberry, red- or blackcurrant or strawberry, which can be extracted by a juicer or liquidizer with a little water and taken frequently for a cooling effect.

Blackcurrant (Ribes nigrum) deserves special attention here. The currants contain high amounts of vitamin C (about 2000mg per kilo), as well as potassium and rutin. Blackcurrant juice should be taken hot as soon as a cold or influenza threatens. So that the vitamins are not destroyed, it is best to add hot water to the juice rather than heating it. It enhances resistance to infection and can be taken with benefit during convalescence.

Fever in Babies

This is treated along similar lines to fever in children. However, a baby should be sponged down more frequently if necessary to keep the fever below 102°F.

You can give the baby boiled water with a few drops of freshly squeezed lemon frequently through the day. You can also give drinks of the juices listed above, diluted with 50 per cent boiled water, either by the teaspoon or in a bottle, as much as the baby will take before putting to the breast. Administer plenty of *camomile tea*.

General Advice

• Babies and children need plenty of love and reassurance when they are ill. They may be frightened or insecure, not understanding why they should suddenly feel so strange. The illness may be simply a cleansing process for the body or its origins may lie further into the psyche, and the illness is unconsciously needed so that the child receives more care and attention which he or she may feel to be lacking. Illness has a habit of disrupting the normal daily routine of the household. Perhaps you could stop awhile and take the opportunity to spend more time with your child and show plenty of love and attention. It may be a wonderful time for the growth and development of the child, of your relationship and even of you.

• Sick children need company and entertainment. Your child will probably love to be read to or told stories. They like plenty to do or look at as they start to recover, so that they do not get bored and unable to resist the temptation to get up before they are fully recovered. At times when parents are busy, books, jigsaws, tapes, the radio and drawing material may help.

• Rest can be anywhere; it does not necessarily have to be in bed. Most children will regulate how much they need to rest by how ill they feel. A child with a fever of 102–103°F will probably simply wish to lie quietly in bed. If the fever is lower they may be happy to lie on the sofa or, if it is warm, to sit out in the garden in the shade. A baby or toddler will probably want to be held and may well cry if put into a pram or cot, unless he or she is really sleepy.

• If your child is in bed, change the sheets frequently and keep a window open slightly to keep the air fresh. You can disinfect the atmosphere by spraying herbal teas or water mixed with essential oils into the room using a plant spray. *Marjoram, wormwood, lavender, thyme, rosemary* and *eucalyptus* can all be used. Alternatively cut half an onion and place it in a bowl in the room to cleanse the atmosphere: change it daily.

• Put loose comfortable night clothes on the child, and use light bedclothes – a duvet is probably better than heavy blankets. Check the temperature at regular intervals, administer remedies regularly where applicable, and watch your child's condition and any changes in it.

• A good gauge of adequate fluid intake is the quantity of urine passed. Most children pass water several times daily when well or ill. If the rate decreases, increase the amount of liquid given. If the child does not feel like drinking more, you can freeze juices or herb teas and produce them as ice lollies, which may be more attractive or acceptable. You can also encourage your child to drink by making their favourite drinks, or giving it in a favourite or special mug or an egg cup, or even on a musical teaspoon! If you still meet resistance you can try distracting from the subject with a story or a game while he or she takes a few sips.

• Delicious drinks can be made with fruits, either in a juicer or a liquidizer, and mixed with water. You can choose your child's favourite fruit, be it strawberries, raspberries, plums, peaches, melon or blackcurrant.

Dehydration

Technically a child with a fever needs to drink at least 3–5fl oz (100–150ml) of liquid for each 2.2lb (kilo) of body weight per day. This should be increased to 7fl oz (200ml) per 2.2lb (kilo) if there is vomiting or diarrhoea. It is best to encourage your child to drink every 15–30 minutes, even if it is only a mouthful. If the urine passed is very concentrated, dark and strong smelling, your child is definitely not drinking enough. If he or she has not passed water for over 24 hours or is persistently drowsy, **call your doctor immediately**. To check for dehydration, gather the skin on the child's abdomen together with your fingers. If it does not spring back quickly when released, it may indicate dehydration.

CHAPTER 9

TREATMENT OF CHILDHOOD ILLNESS

THE RESPIRATORY SYSTEM

While the digestive system derives energy from the food we eat, the respiratory system is responsible for deriving energy from the air we breathe. Through respiration we take in oxygen, the vital ingredient for the metabolism of each cell in the body.

The Indians call the air we breathe *prana* – the breath of life. Not only are we breathing in gases vital for the normal functioning of our cells and tissues, but we are also taking in the energy of the atmosphere, which radiates from the trees and other green plants and, ultimately, from the sun. While we can go without food and water for a few days, we cannot live without air for more than a few minutes.

The respiratory system consists of the nose, throat, larynx, trachea, bronchi and lungs. It is the apparatus by which we take in oxygen, with the lungs acting like a pair of bellows. When we breathe in, the intercostal muscles between the ribs contract, expanding the rib cage, while the diaphragm muscles lower the diaphragm. This causes negative pressure inside the lungs, which thus draws in air, via the nose and trachea, to the lungs. Here the oxygen is taken up by tiny blood vessels (capillaries) into the bloodstream and thence, by the circulatory system, to every cell in the body, where it is used for the metabolism of carbohydrates to produce energy and exchanged for the waste products of metabolism (carbon dioxide and water). When we breathe out, the diaphragm and intercostal muscles relax, pushing the air out and expelling the carbon dioxide and water, which are brought to the lungs via the bloodstream.

Most adults breathe in and out between ten and fifteen times each minute, but a child's respiration rate is much faster than this. Underlying this is the greater need of the infant or child to provide energy to every cell as it functions and multiplies and so to allow the rapid growth and development and high levels of vitality that characterize childhood. A healthy respiratory system is, therefore, vital for the healthy development of every child. However, many children are plagued by respiratory problems, ranging from chronic catarrh to frequent chest infections, which compromise the adequate exchange of oxygen and carbon dioxide in the lungs that is necessary for the health and vitality of the rest of the body.

The origin of respiratory problems may lie in the respiratory system itself, for it is open to the atmosphere via the nose and mouth and so vulnerable to air-borne irritation and infection by viruses, bacteria and other microbes. However, since the respiratory system functions, in conjunction with other pathways of elimination of waste products (the skin, bowels and urinary system), as an organ of elimination, an overload of toxins in the body can mean extra work for the respiratory system, which can cause problems. If waste cannot be properly eliminated via one pathway, the others are overburdened. Constipation, for example, causes a retention of toxins in the bowels and creates an overload of toxic matter to be excreted elsewhere, such as via the respiratory system in the form of catarrh. For this reason the overall health of the child needs to be looked at when respiratory problems are considered.

As long as the blood carries adequate nutrition and oxygen to, and the waste products from, each cell, the normal function of all body tissues should be maintained. To make sure that there is sufficient oxygen breathed in, it is vital that children take plenty of fresh air and exercise every day, and that they breathe properly. Congestion of the respiratory passages with catarrh may lead to breathing through the mouth and shallow breathing, which reduces the amount of oxygen taken in. And what about *fresh* air? Even when breathing is adequate, what about the air we breathe? The pollution in the air – cigarette smoke, carbon monoxide, lead from car fumes and so on – becomes the pollution in our lungs, which is then carried in the blood all around the body. This all has to be borne in mind with respiratory problems, and as much done as possible to reduce our environmental pollution.

The air we breathe, is not only vital to our physiological functioning but also to our more subtle processes. In many cultures and religions the use of the breath is central to spiritual practices, such as yoga and meditation, and traditional movements like Qi Gong and Tai Chi. Correct breathing is also vital for our nerves and muscles to permit relaxation and ensure rest, as well as encouraging a clear, alert mind.

THE UPPER RESPIRATORY SYSTEM: EAR NOSE AND THROAT

Children are more prone to upper respiratory infections – runny noses, sore throats, earaches and coughs – than anything else. Most of these problems are easily treated at home without professional help and, if they are dealt with speedily and effectively, they should not cause complications. In most cases simple dietary measures and herbal remedies, combined with rest and nurture, will suffice, so that antibiotics and other drugs can be kept for more serious conditions for which there is no better alternative.

Nose

As well as being the organ of smell, the nose is a first line of defence against invading organisms. The hairs at the entrance to each nostril and microscopic cilia in the mucous membrane lining further back filter the air. These hairs and cilia act to move forward any foreign matter, dirt, dust or microbes breathed in, which are ejected forcibly by sneezing or blowing. The nose also helps to moisten the air that is breathed in, as it passes over mucus-secreting cells, which is important for the proper exchange of oxygen and carbon dioxide in the lungs. The mucus also acts to protect the delicate linings of the nose.

Sinuses

The spaces or cavities in the bones around the nose are lined with mucous membranes and are

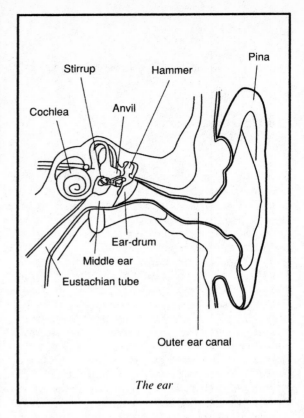

The ear

connected to the nose by small pathways. When the nose is catarrhal or there is an infection in the area, they may become involved, in which case there may be pain around the sinuses and purulent discharge.

Ear

The ear, the organ of hearing and balance, has three different compartments – the outer, middle and inner ear. The outer ear and its canal extend as far as the ear drum, which separates it from the middle ear. The middle ear is connected to the throat by the eustachian tube, which allows passage of air to, and drainage of mucus from, the middle ear, which is necessary for the proper vibration of the ear drum and is, therefore, essential for normal hearing. The eustachian tube is very close to the tonsils and adenoids, which may swell and block the opening of the tube, so preventing air from reaching the middle ear. This predisposes to the development of middle ear infection and explains why so many children have earache and ear infections with upper respiratory ailments.

90

Throat

Like the nose, the mouth and throat are open to the atmosphere and therefore vulnerable to airborne dirt and disease. The lymphatic tissues, the adenoids and tonsils, are vital in the protection of the respiratory tract from irritation and infection. They guard the nasal passages and the throat respectively and, when infection threatens, they swell, as they rally their defences and increase the production of special white blood cells (lymphocytes) to help resolve infection.

THE COMMON COLD

The common cold virus, like any other infection, can thrive only when the conditions are right in the body – the child is tired and a little run down, or there is a tendency to catarrh or to eat too much sugar and junk foods. Babies and toddlers tend to catch colds easily when they are exposed to them because their immune systems are still immature and not as robust as those of older children. However, older children may also catch colds frequently, especially in the winter, when conditions, such as stress, poor diet or living in a polluted, smoky atmosphere affect the immune system so that it is unable to throw off the virus.

A typical cold starts with a sore throat, sneezing and a runny nose. The virus causes irritation of the mucous membranes of the nose, and the rest of the upper respiratory tract, causing them to swell and secrete more mucus in an attempt to dilute the irritant and discharge it from the body. The catarrh that builds up and is then expelled from the body by blowing the nose, provides a useful way for the body to cleanse itself of toxins that have accumulated. For this reason, a cold can be useful – it shows us that the immune system can actually throw off the bad effects of stress and poor diet in a vital way, and should leave the child feeling better for the 'clear-out' afterwards. To this end, it is important not to suppress the body's efforts but to help it in its cleansing work.

As everyone has experienced, swollen nasal passages make breathing difficult, causing mouth-breathing, and they can even close tear ducts, causing runny eyes. Mucus from the nose runs forwards and backwards into the throat, producing a runny nose and often a tickly cough. The adenoids tend to swell,

---

Symptoms of the Common Cold

- ☐ Sore throat and often swollen glands
- ☐ Aches and pains
- ☐ Sneezing
- ☐ Runny nose, watery and copious at first, then thicker and yellow; green if infected
- ☐ Blocked nose, difficulty breathing through nose
- ☐ Runny eyes
- ☐ Tickly cough
- ☐ Blocked or popping ears
- ☐ Often a slight fever
- ☐ Tiredness and often irritability

---

blocking the eustachian tube and causing congestion and popping in the ears. The child may run a slight fever.

To begin with, the mucus is clear and runny. As the cold progresses it may dry up and become thicker and yellow coloured. It can get bacterially infected, and turn purulent and green. This process can take up to two weeks in an infant or toddler, but, as a child's immunity develops, it may be over in a few days, as long as there are no complications.

If any of the symptoms get noticeably worse – if, for example, temperature goes up above 102°F (38.8°C), the popping in the ears turns to constant pain, or an irritating cough becomes more persistent and produces more mucus – prompt action is needed because complications are developing. Also bear in mind that many other infectious diseases begin with cold symptoms before any other characteristic symptoms emerge – the rash with measles, the whoop with whooping cough, for instance.

See also: Middle ear infection, Bronchitis, Sinusitis, Measles, Whooping cough, Sore throat, Pneumonia, Croup, Mumps and Chicken pox.

Herbal Treatment of Colds

There is much variation in the way colds are treated. Some people do nothing and let them take their course, others rush straight to the doctor and are given antibiotics, which are no help anyway for a cold virus, as antibiotics will only affect bacterial infections. When treating children, it is always best to treat them at the first sign of a cold so that the symptoms do not drag on or develop into sinusitis or coughs or worse. This is especially important if the child has a history of catarrhal or chest problems or of asthma. Using herbs, the aim is to support the body's fight against the infection and speed recovery while, at the same time, relieving the often annoying symptoms.

Herbal Infusions

At the first signs, hot herbal infusions sweetened with honey, or flavoured with unsweetened blackcurrant juice or liquorice, can be given.

Boneset This is one of the best remedies to relieve aches and pains, reduce the fever and clear the catarrh quickly.

Elderflowers A great decongestant, an infusion of elderflowers helps to relieve the catarrh.

Yarrow This can be used to increase the circulation, and induce sweating as an aid to the cleansing process. It helps to clear the catarrh, reduce fever and soothe aches and pains.

Peppermint A stimulating decongestant, peppermint helps to clear the catarrhal congestion and reduce fever.

A combination of equal parts of the above taken frequently through the day should see the cold off!

Agrimony, eyebright and golden rod These also help to clear the catarrh.

Eucalyptus, hyssop, pine, rosemary and thyme These all contain volatile oils, which are antiseptic and which stimulate the mucous membranes and help to loosen and clear the mucus congestion.

Camomile This is useful in all children's infections, helping to soothe a fractious child and to induce a healing sleep – nature's way of aiding speedy recovery. This wonderful plant also contains antiseptic volatile oils, which help to resolve the infection, clear the catarrh and reduce fever.

Decoction of Spices

A decoction of spices makes a delicious drink and is also very effective, especially when there is copious catarrh and a very stuffed-up feeling.

½oz fresh ginger (sliced)
1 stick cinnamon
3 cloves
1 teaspoon coriander seeds
Place the ingredients in a pan. Cover with 1 pint (600ml) of cold water. Bring to boil. Cover, simmer for 10–15 minutes and strain. Sweeten with honey or add a slice of lemon if you want. It needs to be drunk as hot as possible.

• If the eyes are particularly affected, *eyebright* can be added to any recipe you choose.

• If there is a sore throat or an irritating cough, soothing herbs – such as *marshmallow, comfrey* or *mullein* – can be added.

• If there is a very painful throat and swollen glands, *cleavers* or *blue flag* can be combined with other herbs.

• Gargles or throat sprays made from pure *lemon juice, raspberry leaf tea, sage tea* with a teaspoon of cider vinegar or tincture of *myrrh* can be used several times a day. Spray bottles are available from most chemists.

• If the catarrh affects the throat or chest and a cough develops, *coltsfoot, hyssop, mullein* and *thyme* can be made into a hot infusion and alternated with the other recipe chosen. *Liquorice sticks* can also be chewed.

• To help fight off the infection, *echinacea* can be added to teas. Alternatively, *garlic* can be taken – one or two perles three times daily or a half to a whole clove of raw garlic chopped into a teaspoon of honey twice a day.

Dosages When you make herbal teas or other recipes to give to children, you have to use your imagination to some extent. The standard dose is only a rough guide. The most important thing is that your child will drink it, so it has to be made to their taste – not so strong that they do not like it and not so weak that the remedy is not effective. There is always a variety of possible remedies for you to choose from, and you may have to experiment a little to find what your children like or, at least, will tolerate. The dosage will also vary according to how much your child wants to drink. If he or she wants sips, give them more frequently than if half a cupful is drunk at a time. You should aim to give between three and six cupfuls a day.

Baths Herbal infusions can be used not only to drink but also to add to bath water and for hand and foot baths, especially if the child is unwilling to drink very much. Here is a useful old recipe for throwing off colds. Mix 1 dessertspoonful of *dry mustard* powder to 2 pints hot water. Soak the feet for 5–10 minutes, twice daily. Cover the head with a hat to increase body heat. *Cinnamon*, *cloves* and *ginger* can be used in the same way.

Inhalations Essential oils can be used as inhalations for children over three years of age. Add between two and five drops of oil to a bowl of boiled water two or three times each day. Putting a towel over the head stops the volatile oils from escaping into the atmosphere. For younger children, the same oils can be used in a vaporizer, which can be especially useful in children's bedrooms at night.

Camomile, *cloves*, *eucalyptus*, *lavender*, *lemon*, *pine* and *thyme* are all antiseptic and help to relieve congestion. They can be used singly or in combination.

Massage and Salves Essential oil of *eucalyptus*, *lavender* or *pine* can be diluted in a base oil (two drops to 5ml) and massaged into the chest, neck, throat or feet or added to bath water. They can also be made into salves using petroleum jelly by mixing ten drops of each into 50 grams of petroleum jelly. Melt the petroleum jelly in a small pan on the stove; when it is liquid, stir in the oils. Pour it into a pot with a good lid, and, when it is cool, seal the lid.

Dietary Treatment of Colds

• In my opinion, it is best to give as little as possible to a coldy child to eat, and let all the energy go to the healing and recovery. If your child is hungry, give vegetables, soups and vegetable juices, fruit and fruit juices, but avoid all dairy produce, meat and grains until the catarrh is cleared. This will probably not

prove difficult, as most children go off their food during a cold.

• Add plenty of antibiotic garlic and onion to their food. Leeks are also useful for the immune system. Foods containing vitamins A and C will help throw off the virus.

• Hot lemon and honey drinks can be given frequently to help clear catarrh and soothe a sore throat.

• Blackcurrant tea, available from health food shops, is delicious and therapeutic for catarrh, infections and fever.

• Supplements of natural vitamin C (chewable tablets of 100mg given three to five times daily), 1 teaspoon cod liver oil and zinc lozenges (5mg three times daily) can be given until the child is quite well again.

To help prevent colds, add plenty of garlic and onions, carrots, watercress and parsley to a diet high in fresh fruit and vegetables. Garlic perles, cod liver oil and vitamin C supplements are useful taken daily as a preventative measure, especially during winter months.

CATARRH

If the lining of the respiratory tract is irritated, it secretes more mucus, which builds up into catarrh. It accompanies infections such as colds, influenza, measles, chicken pox and allergic conditions such as hay fever and asthma.

It is quite common, after a cold, to have catarrh for a few days until the mucous membranes are fully recovered. In some children, however, the catarrhal stage may persist for weeks or it may exist chronically, with or without infection. There are several reasons for this:

• The air passages can be irritated by pollutants in the atmosphere – cigarette smoke, dust, petrol, car exhaust fumes, dry air from central heating and so on.

• A poor diet – the wrong foods, too much milk, sugar and refined carbohydrates or wrong combinations of foods – can cause constipation and putrefaction in the bowel and allow toxins to be circulated in the bloodstream. Mucus or catarrh is one way in which the body can discharge some of its toxic overload.

- Sometimes an allergy to milk (or wheat) causes persistent catarrh, which gives rise to frequent infections – colds, sore throats, chest and ear infections. If your child is particularly prone to these, try omitting *all* milk products from their diet for one or two months. In my experience, a large percentage of children who develop recurrent upper respiratory infections have a milk intolerance. With treatment, this can be dealt with and milk produce slowly reintroduced into the diet. It is always a good idea to give honey with milk, as this helps to break down any excess mucus formed.

- Chronic catarrh can also be due to sinusitis (see below), in which case it will often affect the throat as well as the nose, as the mucus from the infected sinuses runs down the back of the throat. This will irritate the throat, causing a tickly cough, especially when the child is lying down, or constant clearing of the throat.

Herbal Treatment of Chronic Catarrh

- Astringent herbs, such as *elderflower*, *eyebright*, *golden rod* and *plantain*, can be used to tone and heal the mucous membranes and protect them from irritation.

- Herbs with volatile oils are stimulating and help to loosen the sticky mucus, making it easier to blow out through the nose or cough up from the throat. These herbs include *camomile*, *peppermint* and *thyme*, and *eucalyptus*, *ginger* and *hyssop*. Choose one or two herbs from each group and combine them with *echinacea* for low-grade infection and give as a hot infusion, a cupful from three to six times a day.

- Dilute essential oils can be used for inhalations, in vaporizers, in the bath or for local massage of the face, around the nose and sinuses, the throat and chest. Choose from *camomile*, *eucalyptus*, *lavender*, *lemon*, *peppermint* and *pine*.

- Where there are sluggish bowels or the wrong diet, bowel cleansing is recommended for the first week or two of treatment, using *liquorice* or *dandelion root* tea or *linseed* tea. *Garlic perles* or raw *garlic* with honey or salad dressing should be given daily, to clear putrefactive bacteria in the bowel, as well as to help clear the catarrh or sinus infection.

Dietary Treatment of Catarrh

- For the first two or three days of treatment, give the child a light diet consisting largely of fresh fruit and vegetables, vegetable soups, vegetable and fruit juices and herbal teas. For the next two or three weeks, give no sugary foods, no milk or meat and little starchy food. Give plenty of dried fruit, such as prunes, figs, apricots and raisins, to stimulate the bowels.

- Make sure your child drinks plenty, to encourage elimination via the kidneys. Hot lemon and honey drinks are useful to break down the mucus.

- The skin presents a huge surface area available for the excretion of waste products via the pores, through sweating. If this pathway of elimination is not used by vigorous exercise warming the body up and encouraging sweating, more pressure is put on other means of elimination, and this can mean through catarrh. So, make sure your child takes plenty of fresh air and outdoor exercise. You should also make sure there is plenty of fresh air in the house as well, even in winter, keeping windows open, particularly at night. Bowls of water near radiators in centrally-heated houses may help to reduce drying of the atmosphere. An ionizer may also be useful to reduce harmful effects of the atmosphere on delicate mucous membranes.

SINUSITIS

There are four sinuses (cavities containing air) in the head. These can become congested with mucus and inflamed, leading to infection, especially after a sore throat, cold or influenza, but also on a more chronic level for months, if one or more of the passages to the nose which drain the sinuses becomes blocked. Congestion, inflammation and infection of the sinuses is known as sinusitis. This can produce pain and swelling in the face, around the nose and eyes and can cause headaches and even toothache. It is usually accompanied by a blocked nose, occasional purulent phlegm, and dripping of catarrh into the throat, which may cause an irritating cough or a gravelly voice. It rarely occurs in babies, as their sinuses are not fully developed.

> ### Symptoms of Sinusitis
>
> ☐ Pain and swelling in the face, around the nose and over the eyes
> ☐ Headaches
> ☐ Sometimes toothache
> ☐ Blocked nose
> ☐ Yellow-green phlegm
> ☐ Irritating cough in some children
> ☐ Gravelly voice in some children
> ☐ There may be a slight fever

Treatment of Sinusitis

Congestion in the sinuses can be due, like catarrh, to the overproduction of mucus, in an attempt by the body to cleanse itself of toxins that are not being adequately eliminated elsewhere. You can assess if this is the case with your child by checking whether the bowels are sluggish, urination infrequent and how often they do vigorous exercise at school.

● For sluggish bowels use *dandelion root* or *liquorice tea* or *linseed tea*. (See Constipation, page 137, for further advice.)

● Give plenty of liquids to drink to encourage urination. Herbs such as *uva ursi, camomile* and *celery seed* will be helpful here, taken as teas.

● Make sure your child takes plenty of vigorous outdoor exercise. Herbs, such as *yarrow, garlic, ginger, limeflowers* and *cinnamon*, taken in hot teas or hot foods will help to increase sweating and elimination via the pores of the skin.

● Blockage and infection of the sinuses can also be related to overproduction of mucus due to allergy, most often to cow's milk and milk products (see page 94). A diet that reduces mucus is important, and milk, sugar, meat or flour products should be avoided and plenty of fresh fruit and vegetables, seeds, nuts and unrefined oils included. Proteins and carbohydrates should not be eaten in the same meal, nor if possible, should acid fruit be eaten with carbohydrates. This kind of diet needs to be continued until the sinusitis clears, which may take from two to four weeks.

● Herbs with volatile oils not only stimulate the linings of the sinuses, helping to loosen and shift the mucus, but they have antibiotic qualities that resolve the accompanying sinus infection. These include *aniseed, camomile, cinnamon, eucalyptus, fennel, ginger, hyssop, lavender, peppermint, pine, rosemary* and *thyme,* and these can be taken as hot teas, sweetened with honey or flavoured with *liquorice* or *aniseed,* three times a day. They can either be used singly or in combination, blended to suit the child's taste. If your child gets bored with the flavour, you have plenty to choose from to concoct another.

● Essential oils of the same herbs can be used for steam inhalations. Add a few drops of oil to a bowl of hot boiled water. Keep a towel over the head to stop all the air from escaping. Do this morning and night.

Recipe for Inhalant

30 ml friar's balsam (compound tincture of benzoin from the chemist)
20 drops lavender oil
20 drops eucalyptus oil
10 drops pine oil

Add ½–1 teaspoon to a bowl of hot boiled water.

Once the mucus starts to loosen and drain, it should clear fairly quickly. If not, give teas of astringent herbs, such as *agrimony, elderflowers, eyebright* or *golden rod,* or add soothing herbs, such as *comfrey, Iceland moss, marshmallow* or *mullein* to teas, to soothe the irritated mucous membranes of the nose, throat and sinuses.

● For a particularly persistent sinus infection, combined with general tiredness, irritability or being 'off-colour', antibiotic herbs such as *garlic, echinacea, myrrh* or *baptisia* can be used. *Garlic perles,* or *raw garlic* in honey or salad dressings, can be taken two or three times a day, and the other herbs can be added to other infusions.

● You can choose herbs from each group and mix them together to make a pleasant-tasting drink. For example, use equal parts of *echinacea, elderflowers, hyssop, marshmallow* and *peppermint* and add ½–1 teaspoon to a cup of boiling water. Leave for 5–10 minutes, strain and drink hot three times daily.

• Drinks of hot lemon and honey will also help to reduce mucus congestion, while supplements of zinc, vitamin C, *garlic perles* and cod liver oil taken on a regular basis will help to build resistance to infection. (See Immune System, page 70.)

SORE THROAT

The throat may be affected by a variety of infections involving the respiratory tract, either the nose, the sinuses, the mouth or the lungs, as well as by general systemic health. As with all disease, sore throats need to be seen in the wider context of general health and well-being, and not simply relating to the germs involved. An infection will develop only where conditions are right for it to flourish.

• One of the commonest causes of a mild sore throat, which occurs on waking in the morning and disappears after breakfast every day, is central heating causing low humidity. At night during sleep, the mucous membranes of the nose dry out and swell, producing nasal congestion. This causes mouth-breathing, and the low-humidity air irritates the mucous membranes in the throat, causing soreness. This may be easily remedied by placing a vaporizer or humidifier in the bedroom.

• If tonsils, adenoids and other lymph glands in the neck around the throat are swollen and painful, they are fulfilling their role, along with other lymphatic tissue in the body, in defending the body from infection. The tonsils and adenoids are kinds of lymphatic tissue, which produce white blood cells (lymphocytes) to resolve infection and to stimulate immunity and filter toxins from the bloodstream. They are the first line of defence against pathogens in the atmosphere that are inhaled through the nose and mouth. The adenoids are situated at the back of the nose to guard the nasal passages, while the tonsils, at either side of the throat, guard the mouth and trap much of the infection that enters the throat, thereby protecting the lungs and the rest of the body. Removing the tonsils and adenoids should therefore be regarded as a last resort.

• Infections affecting the throat can be either bacterial or viral, although viral infections are the more frequent. Herbs can be used in either instance, but professional help should always be sought when a child runs a fever with an acute sore throat with swollen tonsils. If the infection is bacterial, it is usually the streptococcal bacterium involved, which can sometimes lead to complications such as nephritis and rheumatic fever. In rare cases it could be diphtheria. Throat swabs taken for culture will confirm whether the infection is of a viral or bacterial origin, although there are also some general guidelines for diagnosis. If a child has a sore throat with runny nose or eyes, slight cough or nasal congestion, it is more likely to be viral, but if the child has only a severe sore throat and swollen glands, with or without fever and malaise, but no accompanying upper respiratory symptom, it is more likely to be a streptococcal infection.

• Children will generally tell you that their throat is sore or that it hurts to swallow. A baby is obviously unable to do this, but you will probably notice any difficulty swallowing and if he or she is off their food. To check the throat, ensure that the light is good and gently depress the tongue with a spoon handle and ask the child to say 'aarh'. You will easily determine if the throat is red and the tonsils swollen and infected by the pus on their surfaces. To check for glandular swelling, gently run your fingers down the neck and under the chin. You may find small round swellings like large peas under the skin.

Treatment of Sore Throats

Herbal treatment is always aimed at supporting the lymph glands in their defensive work, while attention should be paid at the same time to the background causes to the infection. (See Immune System and Infectious Diseases, page 70–72).

• For all sore throats, antiseptic herbs such as *echinacea, golden seal, eucalyptus, wild indigo, myrrh, garlic, onion, sage* and *cloves,* can be used to help the immune system.

• These can be combined with remedies that specifically help the cleansing work of the tonsils, including *poke root* (which should only be given in small amounts), *cleavers, marigold* and *golden seal.*

• Tinctures or infusions of, for example, *thyme*, *sage* or *golden seal*, can be used as gargles or sprayed on to the throat with a throat spray.

• Antiseptic oils can be used for inhalation and to disinfect the room.

• Depending on other symptoms involved, extra herbs can be added to your chosen mixture, such as those for fever management – *elderflowers*, *limeflowers*, *camomile* or *mint* – and soothing herbs to relieve the discomfort, such as *mullein*, *marshmallow* and *coltsfoot*.

• Teas can be sweetened with *liquorice* or honey if required.

TONSILITIS

Tonsils are collections of lymphatic tissue found in the throat, and they provide a first line of defence against pollution and infection entering through the mouth and nose. They also act as a filter to poisons in the bloodstream and those draining from the nose and sinuses. In tonsilitis, the tonsils become swollen, inflamed and painful as they respond to an infection, enlarging and increasing their cleansing work in an attempt to throw it off. Because of their protective role, stopping infection from going further into the body, the surgical removal of the tonsils should only be a last resort. When the tonsils are affected, the adenoids will be also.

Tonsilitis can be acute or chronic. *Acute* tonsilitis flares up quickly in response to a viral or a bacterial infection, and it tends to occur when there is low vital energy, too many toxins in the system and a generally congested or catarrhal state of the upper respiratory tract. It frequently accompanies a cold or influenza virus, laryngitis or mumps. If the infection is bacterial, tonsilitis starts suddenly with a severe sore throat and swollen neck glands, often with a fever, but with no or few accompanying upper respiratory symptoms. The streptococcal bacterium involved can, in rare cases, affect the kidneys (causing nephritis) or the heart (in rheumatic fever). Professional help should always be sought when a child runs a fever with a sore throat and swollen glands.

Possible Symptoms of Tonsilitis

☐ Sore throat, often severely painful, causing difficulty in swallowing
☐ On checking the tonsils, you will see that they are swollen and red, and there could be some pus in spots on them
☐ Swollen neck glands, and aching in the neck
☐ There could be fever, with accompanying aches and pains, headache and malaise
☐ When the adenoids are affected, they block the nose, causing mouth-breathing and snoring
☐ There could be catarrh in the nose or throat, and hoarseness if combined with laryngitis
☐ Poor appetite and lethargy
☐ Swollen tonsils can block the eustachian tube and give rise to middle ear infection and earache (see page 102)

Herbal Treatment of Acute Tonsilitis

At the first symptoms, hot infusions can be given, which should include at least *one* herb from each of the following categories:

• Herbs to help the work of the immune system – *echinacea*, *garlic*, *myrrh*, *sage* and *wild indigo*.

• Herbs to support the lymphatic tissue in its cleansing work – *cleavers*, *marigold* and *poke root* (in small amounts).

• Herbs to induce sweating and reduce fever if necessary – *camomile*, *catnip*, *elderflowers*, *limeflowers* and *yarrow*.

• Herbs to tone the mucous membranes and clear the accompanying catarrh and inflammation – *agrimony*, *camomile*, *elderflowers*, *ground ivy*, *plantain* and *raspberry leaves*.

• Herbs to soothe and relieve painful tonsils – *coltsfoot*, *comfrey*, *marshmallow* and *mullein*.

A useful recipe and one that I use frequently

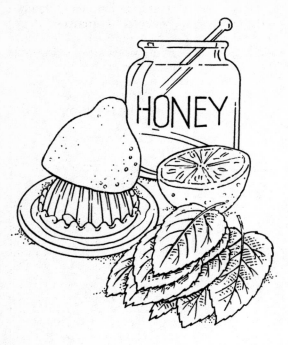

for children with tonsilitis, is to mix equal parts of *cleavers, echinacea, ground ivy, plantain* and *thyme* into an infusion and mix it with ¼ teaspoon *catnip* syrup. Give ½–1 cupful three to six times daily.

Catnip Syrup

To make catnip syrup, heat fresh or dried *catnip* leaves with honey and lemon. Into ½ cup water, 2 tablespoons clear, runny honey and 2 tablespoons fresh lemon juice, chop or crush as many leaves as you can. Put the mixture in a pan on the stove and heat slowly until it is almost boiling. Do *not* boil, but simmer for 5–10 minutes. Leave to cool. Press through muslin (or a wine pressing bag) and store in an airtight bottle in the refrigerator.

At the same time give *garlic* every two hours.

Gargles or throat sprays

These can be made using pure lemon juice or infusions or a teaspoon of tincture diluted in warm water of *camomile, ground ivy, myrrh, sage* or *thyme*. These can be used every two hours if the throat is very painful; otherwise three times a day.

Inhalations

These can be given, using strong infusions or essential oils of *camomile, eucalyptus, lavender* or *thyme*. Friar's balsam could also be used. Put a towel over the child's head if he or she is old enough and allow to inhale for five minutes every few hours. The same oils can be used in vaporizers, diluted for massages or added to water for compresses applied to the throat and neck.

Dietary Treatment of Tonsilitis

A fruit or fruit and vegetable fast, if there is a fever, is recommended for a day or two. Avoid dairy produce, grains and animal produce for a week. Give the child plenty to drink in the form of hot lemon and honey, honey and cider vinegar, herbal teas, fruit juice or carrot juice. Blackcurrant tea or juice (unsweetened) taken hot is excellent for helping to ward off infection and to relieve the sore throat and catarrh. Continue using this after the acute symptoms are gone, as it helps convalescence and increases resistance to further infection.

Supplements of a teaspoon of cod liver oil daily, 100mg natural vitamin C tablets every two or three hours and one or two garlic perles every two hours can be given until the child is well again.

CHRONIC TONSILITIS

In chronic tonsilitis there are recurrent bouts of tonsilitis, between which the tonsils remain swollen. It may be that the tonsils are being overworked by toxins draining from elsewhere, such as chronic catarrh in the sinuses or ears, or by allergic response, very often to milk produce. The child is usually run down from, for example, poor diet, digestive problems, sluggish bowels and pollution in the atmosphere, including passive smoking. Chronic tonsilitis is very often the result of an overuse of antibiotics when treating acute bouts. It could also have an emotional background – the throat area is related to the voice and its use in the expression of emotions and communication. If there are unexpressed or suppressed emotions, such as anger or resentment, these could cause problems around the throat.

It is important that the parents of a child

with chronic tonsilitis assess the deeper causes of the problem, so that it can be completely resolved. This may need to be done with the help of a herbal practitioner. Otherwise, frequent tonsilitis and constantly inflamed or pus-filled tonsils may not be able to continue efficiently with their cleansing work, and other parts of the body may later be affected by the illness.

Treatment of Chronic Tonsilitis

This will follow similar lines to treatment of acute tonsilitis.

• Herbs for the immune system, such as *echinacea* and *garlic*, should be combined with remedies to support the lymphatic system, such as *cleavers* or *poke root* (used only in small amounts), and herbs to tone the mucous membranes such as *ground ivy* and *plantain*.

• In addition, extra herbs, such as *blue flag*, *burdock*, *celery seed*, *echinacea*, *marigold*, *nettles* and *red clover*, need to be used to help the body eliminate toxins and to cleanse the system.

• Gargles or throat sprays using *sage* and *thyme* can be used morning and night.

• Regular massages or compresses, applied to the throat area, can be given, using strong infusions of the herbs used for teas or from essential oils of *rosewood* or *thyme*.

• Make sure the diet contains plenty of fresh fruit and vegetables, nuts and seeds and unrefined oils. Avoid milk produce altogether, preferably for a few months, making sure that you include plenty of other calcium-containing foods in the diet (see page 177). Keep sugar, refined carbohydrates and red meats to an absolute minimum.

• Give supplements of vitamin C, 500mg daily, a teaspoon of cod liver oil, and *garlic perles*, two twice daily, until the problem is resolved.

• Ensure that your child is getting plenty of rest and sleep, regular gentle exercise and fresh air.

• If there are particular emotional difficulties in the family, or at school, it is important to put time aside to talk these over, and allow your child expression of his or her feelings. This can be very healing for everyone.

LARYNGITIS AND CROUP

Mild inflammation and infection of the larynx can spread from infection in the mouth, throat or nose, or from mucus dripping down the throat during a cold. The larynx feels sore and talking can be painful, there is hoarseness and a dry cough, and sometimes a fever. Laryngitis can also occur with tonsilitis or bronchitis, in which case it will be more serious. The child will feel quite ill, there will be a higher fever and malaise. Irritation from a dusty or smoky temperature, too much singing, talking or shouting can also contribute to an inflamed larynx.

Treatment of Laryngitis

• Steam inhalations are very soothing to the larynx and, if essential oils are added to the hot water, their antiseptic and anti-inflammatory properties can bring swift relief. Choose from *camomile*, *eucalyptus*, *lavender*, *pine*, *rosewood* and *sandalwood*. Friar's balsam is also useful.

• The same oils can be used for compresses applied regularly to the throat and chest, or in massage oils or petroleum jelly rubs.

• Herbal infusions can be made using *camomile*, *catnip*, *coltsfoot*, *echinacea* and *marshmallow* flavoured with *liquorice* and sweetened with honey. Give a half to one cupful every two hours.

• *Garlic* can be given every two or three hours. Hot lemon and honey drinks, or blackcurrant tea can be alternated with the herbal tea.

• Keep the air in the room moist, and discourage the child from talking to allow the larynx to recovery quickly.

99

• When the larynx is inflamed, it swells and can go into spasm. In small children the swollen larynx can obstruct the passage of air and cause croup – a barking or whistling sound made as the child tries to breathe through a tense windpipe and past inflamed vocal cords. Babies and small children are particularly prone to croup as their air passages are so small and become easily blocked with mucus when they are inflamed. Croup can be caused by various viral or bacterial infections, including the common cold and bronchitis. The typical pattern begins with a child going to bed with a slightly runny nose. During sleep, mucus runs down the throat, irritating the larynx, causing it to swell and go into spasm. The child wakes up coughing and often struggling to breathe. Frightened by this, the child tenses up, making the situation worse.

If the child breathes very fast, and there is blueness around the face and lips, call the doctor immediately.

Treatment of Croup

Seeing your child having trouble breathing can be very alarming for parents. However, it is important to try to remain calm (at least outwardly) to reassure the child and calm him or her down.

• Sit the child up in bed, which helps breathing anyway, and put a bowl or kettle of steaming water nearby, or take him or her to the bathroom and turn on the hot tap. A steamy atmosphere soothes the air passages, relaxing the spasm in the throat.

• Give *Rescue Remedy* (see Bach Flower Remedies, page 165) to the child (and you if necessary) and *camomile tea* to relax. Open the window a little, to allow the air to circulate.

• Herbs and oils can be added to the boiling water to soothe the inflamed larynx, clear the mucus and relax the spasm. Choose from *birch leaves, eucalyptus leaves, lavender flowers* or *pine needles* and oils of *camomile, eucalyptus, lavender* or *pine*. A few drops of essential oil can be added to water in a plant spray and sprayed into the room, they can be dropped on a damp towel on the radiator or in a bowl of water, or used in a vaporizer, in the bath or for hand and foot baths. They can be mixed with petroleum jelly and rubbed into the chest, throat or back, or used in compresses to apply frequently to the head or chest.

• Infusions, made from any of *camomile, catnip, coltsfoot, horehound, marshmallow* and *wild cherry*, can be given to the child to drink in sips (or in a bottle for a baby).

• A useful recipe for croup, to clear the phlegm and reduce the spasm, is to mix equal parts of *catnip, coltsfoot, cubeb berries, horehound* and *wild cherry* mixed with a pinch of *blood root* if you have it, and flavour them with *liquorice*. Give a tablespoonful or so every 30 minutes until the breathing is better.

• Alternatively, you could use a proprietary brand of antispasmodic drops, giving three or four drops in a little warm water every 15 minutes if necessary. A few drops can be applied to the throat as a linament.

• During the following day or two, give plenty of herbal teas, hot lemon and honey, or a little cider vinegar in a glass of warm water.

• Keep the air in the room moist, and keep the child warm.

• It is important to keep the bowels open to help clear the phlegm; if necessary add more *liquorice* or *senna* to prescriptions for their laxative effect.

• At night, give the child a long hot bath with oils or strong herbal infusions added to the water.

• Rub olive oil, with a few drops of *lavender oil*, into the chest and give a cup of hot herbal tea. If this is done before the child goes to sleep, and air in the bedroom is kept moist, it should prevent the child from waking up with another attack during the night.

• Keep the child on a very light diet, with plenty of fruit and vegetables until the symptoms are completely clear. *Slippery elm powder* mixed with water is very soothing and nutritious. Flavour with honey if you wish.

EAR PROBLEMS

The first part of the ear that sound reaches is the outer ear and its canal, which are separated from the middle ear by the eardrum. The sound waves cause the drum to vibrate, which passes the sound to three tiny ossicles in the middle ear, and from here to the fluid in the cochlea of the inner ear, where sound is carried by the nerves to the brain for interpretation. In addition to the cochlea, in the inner ear are three semi-circular canals bathed in fluid. These are connected to nerve fibres whose function is to indicate the position of the body in space. When this part of the inner ear is disturbed, it causes dizziness and disorientation. The ear is a delicate part of a child's body, and prone to problems because of its proximity to the rest of the upper respiratory tract. The ear, nose and throat are all linked by the eustachian tube, so many colds, sinus and throat infections and catarrhal congestion can lead to the development of earache and ear infections.

EARACHE

Earache can be a very painful condition, which occurs frequently in small children, who are often too young to understand or convey to parents why they are crying, except perhaps to pull at their ear or scratch their face.

Causes of Earache

• It can be due to pain in the throat, gums, teeth or parotid glands (in mumps), which radiates to the ear.

• It can be due to inflammation of the outer ear canal (Otitis externa), with swelling and an irritating discharge; sometimes boils can appear here, which can also be very painful.

• Most commonly, especially in children under six, earache is caused by middle ear infection (Otitis media).

PROBLEMS IN THE OUTER EAR

Objects in the Ear

Small children are very interested in their own bodies and love to investigate small holes. They can poke all sorts of objects into the ear, such as matches, paper clips, hair grips and beads. All tiny things such as these should be kept well out of their reach. If an object such as a bead is pushed in and does not get pulled out, it may be small enough to go unnoticed by either parent until an unpleasant infected discharge appears from the ear. If this occurs, look closely into the ear using a torch if necessary and, if the object is visible and easy to get hold of, then *gently* pull it out. Do *not* try to poke anything into the ear, or insert something in to pull the object out, as the delicate ear is very easy to damage. Take the child to the doctor as soon as possible if the object is stuck.

If an insect gets into the ear, there is a little more you can do. A few drops of water or olive oil will drown the creature and it will float to the surface and emerge from the ear. Do not poke about.

Wax is a normal protective substance secreted by glands in the ear canal, which helps to trap microbes and dirt. If there is too much wax it can create a plug, which blocks sound. Many believe that syringing is the answer. However, the production of wax should perhaps be interpreted as the body's attempt to protect itself from something irritating or potentially harmful, such as excess catarrh in the eustachian tube or a low-grade infection in the middle or outer ear. This needs to be looked into first. Meanwhile, to improve hearing, simply pour warm olive oil into the ear to soften the wax, which, once loosened, will automatically come out of the ear. Syringing may only serve to irritate the ear more, causing it to secrete more wax, and a vicious circle is created.

Infection of the Outer Ear (Otitis externa)

Infection of the outer ear can be caused by:

• An object stuck in the ear
• A boil in the ear canal
• Scratching or fiddling with the ear, which often happens when children have a skin irritation such as eczema in or around the ears
• Chlorine in swimming pools can irritate the skin of children who swim frequently and who do not dry their ears properly

The affected part of the ear becomes red, swollen and painful. There is often itchy, scaly skin and a discharge from the ear, which may smell unpleasant. The infection needs to be treated promptly otherwise it may spread to other parts of the ear. If there is a discharge from the ear, professional advice should be sought, as it may mean a perforated eardrum and a middle ear infection.

Treatment

• First of all, look into the child's ear for signs of irritation or infection, or any foreign object. If there is something in the ear which is easily removed, do so, but do not poke anything into the ear, not even a cotton bud.

• Check the glands and tonsils to see if the earache is caused by another infection.

• Any discharge in the outer ear can be washed away gently with a warm infusion of antiseptic herbs, such as *camomile*, *elderflowers*, *golden seal* or *marigold*, or a few drops of tincture can be used in warm water.

• Drop some warm olive oil with a few drops of essential oil (two drops to a teaspoon of oil) into the ear canal before bed and plug gently with a little cotton wool. Use *camomile* or *lavender* or pierce a *garlic perle* and squeeze it into the ear.

• Try to prevent your child from scratching the ear, and make sure that the hands and fingernails are clean, in case they fiddle with the ear when asleep or out of sight.

• Do not let water from the bath or shower into the ear until it is better. Swimming is not a good idea until then.

MIDDLE EAR INFECTION

Infection from the nose or throat can be carried, via the eustachian tube, into the middle ear and, because this tube is relatively short in babies and young children, they are particularly prone to infection. Catarrh and swollen tonsils or lymph glands in the throat can block off the opening of the eustachian tube into the

---

Possible Symptoms of Middle Ear Infection

☐ Pain in the ear and the area around it
☐ Deafness on the affected side
☐ Fever and often great distress
☐ Pus discharged from the ear
☐ Inflamed and swollen tonsils
☐ Swollen glands
☐ A baby or toddler will rub or pull the ear, and will cry or even scream, and seem generally off-colour

---

throat, creating stasis and a build-up of catarrh in the middle ear, producing infection.

The first signs are acute earache, causing great pain and crying, followed often by deafness in the affected ear. There may be a fever and, as pus forms behind the eardrum, the pressure intensifies, which can lead to perforation of the eardrum as a tiny hole is made to allow discharge of the purulent mucus. This immediately relieves the pressure and the pain, but does not necessarily mean that the infection has cleared.

If you suspect that your baby or child has a middle ear infection, consult your practitioner, as this is a potentially serious condition.

If the eardrum perforates once or twice, healing should be quick and thorough and no further problems need develop. If earache with infection occurs frequently, causing perforation, this may leave permanent scarring of the eardrum, which limits the ability of the ear drum to vibrate carrying sound to the middle and inner ear. This can lead to impairment of hearing.

Unresolved infection can spread to the bony structure behind the ear (mastoid process) or into other parts of the head. Because of this risk, all ear infections need to be treated promptly, and any tendency to recurrent infection resolved. Frequent antibiotics are not the answer, as they do not address the underlying conditions predisposing to infection.

Glue Ear

This is a chronic condition of the middle ear in

which it fills up with a thick, sticky discharge that impairs hearing. It is related to frequent upper respiratory infections – sinus, throat and middle ear infections – and is generally found where there are chronically enlarged tonsils, adenoids and lymph glands in the throat and neck area, which can block the eustachian tube. This can explain much of the build-up of mucus in the middle ear, as the blocked eustachian tube does not allow normal drainage.

The orthodox treatment for glue ear is the surgical insertion of grommets into the child's ear. These are little tubes, which allow drainage from the middle ear, and they can be helpful in the short term as they minimize problems with deafness. However, in the long term, there is no clear indication that they are any better in terms of the scarring to the eardrum, than frequent ear infections with some perforations. Certainly, if surgery and general anaesthetics can be avoided, so much the better. The answer lies in constitutional treatment of the child, looking at causes and not just symptoms.

Treatment of Acute Middle Ear Infection

• As long as there is no pus in the ear and the drum has not perforated, a few drops of warmed oil can be dropped into each ear, and plugged with cotton wool. Oils can be chosen from the following:

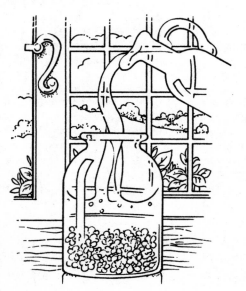

Mullein Oil This is made from yellow mullein flowers, picked in the summer when fresh, placed in a jar and covered in olive oil. Leave the jar on a sunny window sill for two weeks and then press through muslin. Store in a cool place.

Garlic Oil You can either prick a garlic capsule (warmed in your hands) with a pin and squirt the oil into the ear or you can press fresh garlic and mix it with some olive oil. Leave it to macerate for an hour or more, press and then draw some *warmed* oil up into a dropper and put a few drops in each ear.

St John's Wort Oil This is made in the same way as mullein oil, using freshly picked yellow St John's wort flowers.

Essential Oils Any of the following can be used, diluted (two drops of essential oil to a teaspoon of olive oil): *camomile, eucalyptus, lavender* or *rosewood*. These can also be massaged into the area around the ears, neck and throat. Hot compresses can be applied directly to the ears and neck area to ease the pain. Use a few drops of essential oil to a bowl of hot water. Repeat frequently as required. Foot baths can be used with the same mixture.

A few drops of tincture of *myrrh* or *golden seal* can be added to oils to drop in the ears.

Recipe for Eardrops

This recipe can be made up and kept in the medicine cupboard.

> 15 drops golden seal tincture
> 5 drops lobelia (or myrrh) tincture
> 15 drops eucalyptus oil
> 5 drops pasque flower tincture
> 15 drops lavender oil

Mix in 30 ml of olive oil or almond oil. Use two drops of the warmed mixture in each ear.

• A hot-water bottle, held against the painful ear, can also be soothing for many children.

• Teas or tinctures can be given frequently to help relax the child, soothe the pain, combined with remedies to resolve the infection and reduce the congestion. Choose at least one from each group:

☐ Antiseptic herbs – *camomile*, *echinacea*, *hyssop* and *peppermint*.

☐ Relaxant herbs – *camomile*, *pasque flower* and *skullcap*.

☐ Herbs to reduce catarrhal congestion – *elderflowers*, *golden rod* and *ground ivy*.

● To help reduce fever if it is high, add *limeflowers* to your prescription. A remedy combining some of these herbs should be used at the first sign of earache, and repeated frequently, every hour or two if necessary. Use equal parts of *camomile*, *echinacea*, *elderflowers*, *hyssop* and *limeflowers*, sweetened with honey if you wish.

● In addition, give the child *garlic perles*, one every two hours during the acute stage. As the pain diminishes and the child seems better, give them three times daily until all signs of infection are gone and the child is quite well again.

● Avoid giving solid food until the acute condition has cleared, but make sure you give plenty to drink – water, fruit juice, herbal teas, carrot juice, onion and garlic juice, but no milk produce.

Treatment of Recurrent Middle Ear Infection and Glue Ear

● If your child is prone to ear infection or has glue ear, it is important to treat the underlying conditions at the root of the problem and not just address the acute infections when they arise. Since chronic ear problems are largely related to throat, tonsil, nose, sinus and catarrhal problems, these need to be resolved, and the immune system strengthened through the use of herbs and diet (see page 70).

● Passive smoking has been found to be closely related to the incidence of glue ear, so make sure that the child has plenty of fresh air and is kept away from smoky or polluted atmospheres as far as possible.

● Avoid foods that are mucus-forming – milk produce, refined carbohydrates, excess wheat and sugar, for example – and make sure that the child eats plenty of fresh fruit and vegetables, and zinc-containing foods (see page 178).

● Give *garlic* every day, either in foods, as juice or in perles, which you can give at night if you are concerned about the more anti-social aspects of garlic's odour.

● Drinks of lemon and honey or cider vinegar and honey will help to clear the mucus and to strengthen the immune system.

● Supplements of cod liver oil, 200–500mg natural vitamin C and a children's multi-mineral and vitamin should be given daily (see Immune System, page 71).

● Children with recurrent upper respiratory and ear infections frequently suffer from chronic catarrh combined with chronically enlarged tonsils and glands in the neck. In many cases this is caused by an allergic reaction to milk produce or sometimes to wheat. It is best to omit all milk produce from the diet, initially for one or two months, if your child suffers from these problems. During this time you can use herbs to help resolve the condition and, at the end of this period, you can reassess the situation. Very often, within the first week or two, a virulent infection arises, which represents the body's reaction – throwing off toxins – and preferably this should not be suppressed with antibiotics. After this there should be signs of improvement: infections should develop much less frequently and, when they do, they should be much milder. If you see some positive change after the first two months, persevere with the milk-free diet for a couple more months and give your child's immune system a proper opportunity to recover. If the child seems well after this, you can (while continuing with the herbal treatment) start to reintroduce small amounts of milk produce – goat's yoghurt initially – once a week or so. If all seems well, you can gradually give it more frequently, and slowly return milk to the diet. Should an infection develop, you have probably gone too far. Withdraw the milk produce again until the symptoms are completely clear, and then start re-introducing again, but this time more slowly. It may be that you need to keep milk produce to a minimum for the best part of a year.

● Herbal remedies need to be given during this time to strengthen the immune system and to help clear catarrhal congestion in the nose, sinuses and throat. Check the tonsils and lymph glands in the neck to see if they are inflamed or swollen, and, if so, add herbs to your chosen prescription for the lymphatic system (see Tonsilitis page 97).

☐ Herbs for the immune system – *camomile, echinacea, hyssop, liquorice, peppermint* and *wild indigo.*

☐ Herbs to clear the catarrh – *camomile, elderflowers, eyebright, golden rod* and *hyssop.*

☐ Herbs for the tonsils and lymph glands – *cleavers* and *marigold.*

Choose one or two herbs from each group and combine them together as an infusion. Give a cupful three times daily.

● Dilute essential oils can be massaged regularly around the nose, throat and ears, and steam inhalations can be given daily using *camomile, eucalyptus, lavender* or *rosewood.*

● Hot compresses can be applied to the nose, ears and throat, and hand and foot baths can be given regularly using the same oils.

● At the first sign of a cold, start to treat the ears with drops, and give the remedies for acute ear infections to help prevent the infection affecting the middle ear (see page 102). Keep the neck, throat and ears warm at all times, and dress the child up well to go outside in cold winter air.

● See also: Tonsilitis, Catarrh, Sinusitis and Immune System.

THE LOWER RESPIRATORY SYSTEM

The air we take in through our nose and mouth travels down the windpipe (trachea). In the chest this divides into two main bronchi, one going into each lung. In the lung, each bronchus divides many times into air tubes, which become smaller and smaller until they end up as bronchioles. These lead into microscopically tiny groups of air sacks (alveoli), which resemble a bunch of grapes. They are surrounded by a fine network of tiny blood vessels, which take up the oxygen from the alveoli and carry it around the body. These blood vessels also bring carbon dioxide, the waste product of oxygen metabolism, to be taken up by the alveoli. From here, it is breathed out via the lungs.

Each part of the respiratory tract can develop inflammation or infection: tracheitis (inflammation of trachea), bronchitis (inflammation of bronchi), bronchiolitis (inflammation of bronchioles), pneumonia (inflammation of alveoli) and broncho-pneumonia (inflammation of both bronchi and alveoli).

COUGHS

A cough, nature's way of cleansing the air passageways, is a reflex response to anything that blocks the throat or bronchial tubes, whether it be an irritant inhaled from the atmosphere, a piece of food going down the wrong way or an infection causing irritation and phlegm. For this reason it is a mistake to take proprietory cough mixes, which act to suppress the cough reflex, since they prevent this protective action by the body and predispose to infection.

Coughs can be dry and irritating, or they can be loose and productive – that is, the coughing produces mucus, which has been loosened from the mucous membranes and excreted in this way. If it is swallowed (as it is normally by a child) it will be processed by the digestive tract and excreted via the bowels.

The irritation in the throat or chest which produces a *dry* cough may be caused by:

● Mucus from infected sinuses (see page 94)

● Mucus draining from the back of the nose during a cold or with catarrh, which trickles down and irritates the throat

● Chemicals in the atmosphere – passive smoking, paint fumes, and so on

● A foreign body in the air-passages – a piece of bread, for instance

● Nervousness causing constriction in the throat area

It may also be related to a need for more attention or to another infection, such as middle ear infection (see page 102), tonsilitis (see page 97) or croup (see page 99).

If a child has a dry hacking cough, which cannot be relieved, or causes wheezing, breathing difficulties (gasping for breath, rapid or laboured breathing) or blueness around the lips, contact your doctor immediately.

A *loose* productive cough is caused by inflamed bronchial tubes producing excess mucus, either because of infection, such as bronchitis (see page 107), or whooping cough (see page 113), or an allergy such as asthma (see page 116).

Congestion, irritation and infection in the chest, as elsewhere in the respiratory tract, can be related to toxins in the bowel, poor circulation via other pathways (skin, bowels and urine), lowered vitality, poor diet, lack of fresh air and exercise, insufficient sleep, or stress.

• When the vitality of a child is already lowered, it is easy for the child to become affected by changes in the weather, from warm to cold or from dry to damp, and to go down with a cold or cough, and it will be blamed on the weather, or the child getting chilled, and the more long-term causes may be ignored. It is important to consider both when treating your child.

• After immunizations, the child's immune system may be struggling to cope with the introduced infections and will not be so robust in warding off other infections going around – a child is often prone to a cold or cough at this time, frequently coupled with a fever and malaise.

Preventing Coughs

• General health and vitality is the key to warding off all disease, including coughs. Preventative measures are the best approach, so that, when winter colds and coughs are rife, your child can withstand the majority of them.

• Encourage your child to take plenty of outside exercise – take him or her out for regular walks or games in the garden, and try to avoid too much sitting around in over-heated houses.

• Always make sure the child wraps up well when going from a warm house to freezing winter air outside, which can put quite a strain on the body and predispose to hard croupy coughs, which can often cause breathing difficulties.

• Mucus-producing foods are best kept to a minimum during the winter months, particularly cow's milk products, sugar and refined carbohydrates. Should a cold or cough develop, omit these completely from the diet.

• A child who is tired and run down, who has been under pressure at school or doing too much, or who does not sleep well, is bound to be more prone to infection. A balance of work and play, activity and relaxation is essential.

• Emotional factors also play a considerable part (grief is the emotion which is connected to the lungs), and this can be related to moving from one school to another, one house to another, from loss of total attention once a baby brother or sister is born, or through parents arguing or divorcing, for example. If you feel that emotional stress plays a part, use supportive measures for the nervous system (see page 125) even before any physical symptoms arise.

Different Types of Cough

The herbal treatment of coughs will depend entirely on the type of cough a child has.

1. **A cough with a fever** may accompany an infection. The infection usually comes on suddenly, there may be a sore, inflamed throat, a catarrhal nose with a cough that is dry and harsh, and can keep the child awake at night.

2. **A cough with catarrh.** There may be a lot of catarrh in the nose or throat. The catarrh starts watery but then thickens as the infection resolves. The child coughs up lots of mucus and is worse at night when lying down, as the tubes become clogged. This kind of cough can also start suddenly, and the child may feel cold and shivery.

3. **A dry, irritating or croupy cough** accompanies laryngitis, croup and tracheitis. It often starts at night with coughing bouts, during which it is hard for the child to draw air. The coughing may make the throat or trachea sore and the child distressed or irritable.

4. **An intermittent, chronic cough** can

continue in between acute infections. There may be lethargy or debility, poor appetite, thick phlegm in the chest, and swollen neck glands. They may have a generally catarrhal condition.

TRACHEITIS

Inflammation and irritation of the trachea produces symptoms that are similar to laryngitis and croup (see pages 99). It usually involves a viral infection, which often spreads from the upper respiratory tract, and produces hoarseness, a hacking dry cough and soreness in the chest. There is not generally a fever.

Follow the treatment for a *dry* cough.

BRONCHITIS

Inflammation of the mucous membrane lining the bronchial tubes is known as bronchitis.

Acute bronchitis can develop from a cold or sore throat, or as a secondary infection – in measles (page 161) and whooping cough (page 113), for example. It can involve either a viral or bacterial infection and, sometimes, a fungal infection, which causes the mucous membranes to swell and produce more mucus. This leads to coughing, in an attempt to clear the airways of congestion, and may make breathing difficult. There can be rapid breathing and sometimes wheezing.

Initially the cough will be dry and irritating, often making the chest sore. After a few days, the cough loosens and green or yellow phlegm is brought up. You may not see this as young children tend to swallow the phlegm, but you will hear the phlegm rattling in the chest and gurgling when the child coughs to clear it. If a child swallows a lot of phlegm, it may cause vomiting at the end of a coughing bout. It is best to encourage the child to cough up and spit out the phlegm. If they are too young, it is a good idea to hold them face down over your lap as they cough, which will make it easier to spit out.

As the body rallies its defences to throw off the infection, the temperature goes up and, naturally, the child will feel unwell and will not want to eat. The child should be kept warm and calm, and in bed for as long as possible, propped up with extra pillows if necessary to

---

Possible Symptoms

Acute Bronchitis

☐ A cough that starts dry and hacking and then, in a few days, produces sticky sputum, either green or yellow
☐ Raised temperature
☐ Loss of appetite
☐ General malaise
☐ Vomiting after coughing
☐ Rapid breathing or wheezing

Chronic Bronchitis

☐ Intermittent coughing
☐ Much phlegm, usually white or yellow
☐ Wheezing or coughing on exertion such as running
☐ General lethargy
☐ Aggravation from damp atmosphere, fog or dust
☐ There may be other signs of upper respiratory congestion – stuffy nose, congested sinuses, enlarged tonsils or lymph nodes and so on – indicating in many cases intolerance of milk produce.

---

ease breathing. Fresh air in the room is important – open a window, but make sure the child is not in a draught. Try to keep pollution, such as cigarette smoke, as far away as possible.

If the fever goes above 102°F (38.8°C) you can lower it with tepid sponging and giving herbal teas (see Fever Management, page 85–8). Encourage the child to drink, to prevent risk of dehydration, but do not give cough suppressants as the mucus needs to be coughed up and cleared.

Consult the doctor immediately if there are breathing difficulties or the child is distressed, there is any sign of blueness around the lips or tongue, the child draws the chest in sharply with each breath or the child becomes lethargic (from dehydration).

Bronchitis can often occur in a *chronic* form. This may develop after repeated bouts of acute bronchitis, by which time the vitality of the child is considerably lowered and the child is not able to throw off the infection in a robust way. In this case, it is most important to look closely into the child's constitution and background factors causing this low state of health – diet, exercise, allergies and the child's emotional environment. In chronic bronchitis there will be a low-grade infection or inflammation of the bronchial tubes, causing intermittent coughing and general debility.

If your child has a chronic cough, it may be that an allergy to certain foods or environmental pollutants is to blame (see Allergies, page 67).

If you think your child may have bronchitis consult your practitioner.

BRONCHIOLITIS

Inflammation of the bronchioles, the smaller tubes that branch from each bronchus, occurs mostly in infants, sometimes in small toddlers. There is usually a viral infection that causes the walls of the tiny bronchioles to swell. When this occurs in the much larger bronchus, it cuts down the airway slightly but, in the bronchioles, it may actually halve the amount of space through which the air has to travel. It can, therefore, cause varying degrees of respiratory distress, depending on how much of the lung tissue is involved in the infection.

Symptoms of Bronchiolitis
- ☐ Rapid breathing
- ☐ Wheezing
- ☐ Difficulty breathing in and out
- ☐ Intermittent cough, which is loose and productive

Call your doctor immediately if your baby is wheezing and has moderate to severe breathing difficulty. The baby may need to be kept in hospital for observation or treatment. It may be necessary to analyse blood oxygen levels and to support fluid intake or nutrition with an intravenous drip.

PNEUMONIA

Pneumonia involves inflammation and infection of the lungs, usually by a virus or bacteria.

Symptoms of Broncho-pneumonia

- ☐ After an initial infection, the child may appear better but then develop a cough and a fever; this can be low grade in some cases and high in others
- ☐ In many cases the child need not be very ill, unless there is a high fever, in which case they will want to stay in bed and there may be headache, shivering and malaise
- ☐ It starts with a dry cough, which then becomes more moist and productive; yellow-green or rust-coloured phlegm may be coughed up
- ☐ There may be soreness, rawness or pain in the chest, particularly when the cough is dry

---

Sometimes it can involve a fungus, or may be caused by the inhalation of irritant vapours or chemicals or by a foreign body, such as food or pus, which has carried microbes into the lungs.

In children, pneumonia occurs mostly as a sequel to another respiratory infection, such as cold, influenza, whooping cough or bronchitis, or to another illness, such as measles, which spreads to the lungs. This is known as broncho-pneumonia. It is more likely to happen when a child has not rested sufficiently during the former illness or when treatment has been aimed at suppressing rather than enhancing the body's healing efforts in throwing off the infection by the use of, for instance, cough suppressants. The invading micro-organisms can reach the alveoli of the lungs only when all the previous natural defences have been lowered. In broncho-pneumonia there are patches of infection scattered around both lungs.

Lobar pneumonia can occur suddenly without warning and, in older children, where there is no other infection. Here, one or more lobes of the lung has become infected, usually by pneumococcus bacteria. When both sides are affected, this is known as double pneumonia. This can be a serious infection and is usually treated promptly by antibiotics.

Several factors can predispose to pneumonia, an infection that indicates that the natural defences of the respiratory system are significantly compromised. These include the effects

Symptoms of Lobar Pneumonia

☐ There is usually high fever, malaise, shivering and headache

☐ There is a persistent hacking cough and sometimes chest pain in the early stages

☐ Within a few days the cough becomes productive

☐ There may be rapid breathing or difficulty breathing

of lifestyle – poor diet, lack of fresh air and exercise, pollution (from passive smoking, for example). It may also occur if a child is weakened by other pathology – cystic fibrosis, for instance – or poor nutrition as in malabsorption or if the lungs have been weakened by chronic problems, such as asthma, whooping cough or measles.

The alveoli of the lungs react like the rest of the respiratory system when irritated: they fill up with fluid, in this case exudate from the surrounding blood vessels. Now, therefore, instead of containing air, the affected alveoli are full of fluid, which reduces the available space in the lungs for breathing and exchange of oxygen and carbon dioxide. This causes shortness of air and produces breathing difficulties.

If you think your child has pneumonia, consult your practitioner. If there is a high fever or severe breathing difficulties, with flaring of nostrils, and heaving of the chest with each breath in the effort to breathe, call your doctor immediately.

Treatment of Coughs

Treatment for Cough with Fever

The herbal treatment of coughs is always aimed at assisting the body in its own healing process, helping the chest to clear itself of phlegm, inflammation and infection while, at the same time, using herbs to enhance the immune system.

Bronchitis and pneumonia produce coughs with a fever, as the body tries to throw off the infection. The fever tends to be at its highest while the cough is still dry and harsh, and comes down as the child perspires and the cough becomes looser and more productive.

● Herbs to help the body fight the infection and resolve the inflammation in the chest include *echinacea, elecampane, eucalyptus, garlic, hyssop* and *thyme*. One or two of these can be combined in a tea with other herbs to help induce perspiration and bring down the fever. Choose from *camomile, catnip, elderflowers, hyssop, limeflowers, pleurisy root* and *yarrow*.

● To help loosen and expel the mucus from the throat and chest and to soothe the irritated bronchial tubes, you can add an expectorant herb to the mixture, such as *coltsfoot, comfrey, Irish moss, liquorice, marshmallow, mugwort* or *mullein*, which are particularly soothing for a dry cough, or *angelica, aniseed, elecampane, horehound, hyssop* or *thyme*, which are more stimulating for a productive cough.

Hyssop Syrup

2 handfuls of flowering stems and leaves
1 pint (600ml) water
1lb (500g) brown sugar

Pour the boiling water over the hyssop in a teapot and leave to infuse overnight. Pour into a pan and add the sugar. Heat gently until the sugar is dissolved. Boil hard for 5 minutes. Skim. When cool, pour into dark bottles with screw tops or corks. Store in the refrigerator. Give two teaspoonfuls from three to six times daily. This also makes a delicious drink and can be used regularly as preventative medicine. You can also pour it over fruit salads.

● A useful recipe, which I have found effective on many occasions, is a tea of equal parts of *coltsfoot, hyssop, limeflower* and *mullein*. Flavour with a little *liquorice* and honey if you like. This needs to be taken frequently through the day – as much as four or six cupfuls to be taken overall – either as sips as frequently as possible by toddlers and small children or in larger amounts by older children.

● This can be alternated with *garlic*, either given as perles every two hours, or as a honey, a useful way to give garlic to children. To make garlic honey cover four cloves of sliced or chopped garlic with 3fl oz (100ml) of runny honey. Leave overnight and then strain off the juice. Give in teaspoon (5ml) doses several times a day. The honey itself has natural anti-biotic qualities.

• If the fever is high, use herbal teas separately to bring down the fever, and give them as frequently as you can. Use the same infusion when tepid to sponge the child down (see Fever Management, page 85–8).

• Essential oils can be used for inhalations, baths, chest rubs, hand and foot baths and massage. Choose from *eucalyptus*, friar's balsam, *lavender*, *pine* and *thyme*.

Within a few hours of treatment in acute chest infections with fever, you should begin to see some improvement. The child should perspire, and the visible signs of fever – such as red cheeks and hot skin – diminish. The harsh cough should become easier and more productive, and the child should feel much better in itself. The child should be watched carefully and all changes in his or her condition assessed. If the fever persists and the cough does not improve, consult your practitioner.

Treatment of Catarrhal Cough

Once a dry, irritating cough has become more loose and productive, the phlegm needs to be cleared from the chest. A catarrhal cough can arise not only in the above circumstances – that is, after a dry cough with fever – but also with a cold, sore throat or influenza, which produces copious catarrh. In this case, the cough may start fairly suddenly, and the child may feel cold and shivery and look pale.

Herbal treatment is aimed at clearing the mucus from the chest and at helping the immune system to fight off the infection and to warm and stimulate the child's system to enable it to resolve the symptoms.

• Several herbs have antiseptic volatile oils in them. These are warming and/or stimulating and are very useful in helping to loosen and expel the mucus from the throat and chest. Choose from *aniseed*, *cinnamon*, *fennel*, *ginger*, *hyssop* and *thyme*. These should be taken as hot teas, three to six cupfuls a day and, since some of them, such as the *cinnamon* and *ginger* are fairly strong tasting, they need to be made to

taste – not so weak that they are not effective but not so strong that the child cannot take them. They can be combined with other herbs such as *coltsfoot* and *horehound* to help clear the phlegm.

Essence of cinnamon can be bought from chemists or herbal suppliers, and it is very useful for persistent coughs and catarrh. Use $\frac{1}{2}$ teaspoon (2–3ml) in a little warm water three to six times a day.

• *Elecampane root* tea, with a small amount of *ginger* and *liquorice* and sweetened with honey, is pleasant tasting and wonderfully effective, particularly when there is a chest infection with phlegm.

• Alternatively, you can use equal parts of *thyme* and *sage* tea spiced with a little powdered *ginger*, *cloves* and *nutmeg*.

• Essential oils can be used for baths, inhalations, massaged into the throat, chest, back and feet, or used as hand and foot baths. Choose from *cinnamon*, *clove*, *eucalyptus*, *ginger*, *lavender*, *pine* or *thyme* or use camphorated oil or friar's balsam which are available from chemists.

• *Garlic* can be taken as perles or in honey every two hours in the acute phase.

Treatment of Dry Cough

A dry, irritating or hacking cough can accompany laryngitis (see page 99) and tracheitis (page 107), which develop usually from an infection in the nose or throat. Mucus dripping down the throat can be responsible for the inflammation, but so can irritation from pollution in the atmosphere, such as dust and smoke, or overuse of that part of the body – by speaking, shouting or singing. The phlegm produced in a dry cough is sticky and scanty and hard to cough up. The swollen larynx in laryngitis, coupled with the sticky phlegm, can obstruct the passage of air, particularly in babies and small children, and lead to croup (see page 99).

• A dry cough needs to be soothed and loosened by herbs with relaxing and demulcent properties, which also help to expel the loosened mucus. You can use any of the following

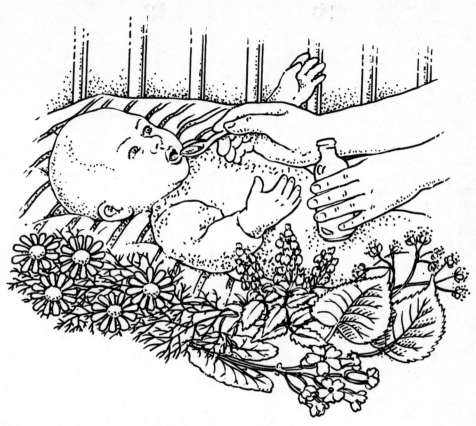

in an infusion or syrup – *coltsfoot, comfrey, linseed, liquorice, marshmallow, mullein* or *wild cherry bark.*

● If the child becomes distressed during the coughing bouts, which can last up to a few minutes each time, this may make the cough worse. Use more relaxing herbs, added to the mixture, which will also help the child to relax and sleep at night, when a dry cough tends to be worse. Useful herbs include: *camomile, catmint, cowslip flowers* and *limeflowers.*

● You can also use Dr Bach's *Rescue Remedy* (see page 167); add a few drops in a drink when necessary.

● As the cough improves it will begin to soften and the phlegm will become looser and easier to expel. You can now give the child expectorant herbs, to help the cough to be more productive, such as *angelica, aniseed, blood root* (in small amounts), *coltsfoot, elecampane, horehound, hyssop* and *thyme.*

Thyme Syrup

To make thyme more palatable for small children, make thyme syrup, which is wonderful for coughs, sore throats and whooping cough. Take three handfuls of finely chopped thyme, cover them with runny honey and leave to macerate for a few hours. This will keep indefinitely. Alternatively, infuse one handful of chopped thyme in one cup of boiling water, until cool. Strain and add honey. This should be kept in a refrigerator and consumed within a few days. Give 1 teaspoon (5ml) of either three or four times daily.

Angelica Syrup

This is very good for irritating dry coughs and sore throats. Pour two cups of boiling water over two handfuls of grated angelica root. Add $\frac{1}{2}$ cup of runny honey and $\frac{1}{4}$ cup of lemon juice. Cover and leave to stand until cold. Strain and bottle. Store in a refrigerator and use within three days. Take 1 teaspoon (5ml) three or four times daily.

Another useful recipe for dry coughs is to add 1 teaspoon (5ml) of a mixture of *aniseed*, *coltsfoot*, *horehound*, *mullein* and *wild cherry* to each cup of boiling water. Give this three to six times daily. Sweeten with honey if you wish.

● Any of the above herbs can be used as strong infusions to add to bath water, especially for babies and small children, who will find it difficult to drink the tea. You can also use them for hand and foot baths, and hot compresses applied to the chest and throat.

● Essential oils can also be used in the bath, for hand and foot baths, steam inhalations, vaporizers and massage. Choose from *camomile*, *eucalyptus*, friar's balsam, *lavender*, *pine* and *thyme*.

● Dry, croupy coughs respond well to steam and to humid atmospheres. You can make the room more humid by hanging a wet towel on a radiator or near a heater, and you could put essential oils on it.

● Frequent drinks of lemon and honey can also be given, to soothe the tickly cough.

● *Garlic perles*, juice or honey should be given regularly three times a day until the child is completely recovered.

● If a baby is having trouble bringing up the phlegm during a coughing fit, place the baby over your knee and gently pat him or her on the back. Massage the back in this position with dilute oils.

● If a child is very troubled at night, prop him or her up in bed with two or three pillows, to stop the mucus from irritating the throat and chest so much.

Treatment of Chronic Cough

Chronic coughs can hang on after an acute infection if the child's vitality is lowered and has not been sufficient to throw off the illness completely. This can happen if the child has not rested sufficiently or if the acute infection was not treated correctly. Often it will arise if the child has been given antibiotics. Alternatively, it can develop after immunizations,

notably whooping cough and polio. In any chronic condition the background to the lowered vitality always needs looking into, whether it is caused by poor diet, lack of fresh air and exercise, emotional problems or overuse of antibiotics. It could also be related to pollution or allergy (see Immune System, page 61).

Herbal treatment needs to include remedies to enhance the immune system, such as *echinacea*, *garlic*, *hemp agrimony* and *wild indigo*, as well as general tonics for convalescence, including *borage*, *cleavers*, *dandelion root*, *marigold*, *nettles* and *red clover*.

● There may be a lot of mucus in the chest, which can be expelled with the help of expectorant herbs such as *aniseed*, *coltsfoot*, *elecampane*, *horehound*, *hyssop*, *liquorice*, *mullein* and *thyme*. This may mean that a chronic intermittent cough can seem worse for a day or so – more frequent and more productive – but this should be a positive sign, as the vitality of the child increases to throw off the illness.

● If there are swollen tonsils and neck glands, be sure to include in your remedy herbs for the lymphatic system, such as *cleavers*, *marigold* or *poke root* (which should be given only in small amounts).

● A useful recipe for a chronic cough is to use equal parts of *aniseed*, *borage*, *coltsfoot*, *echinacea* and *hyssop*. Flavour with *liquorice*, or sweeten with honey, and give a cupful three times daily.

● *Coltsfoot tea* is always *the* remedy of choice in a chronic cough, as it contains bitter tonics as well as being soothing and expectorant. It is best sweetened with honey. Hot lemon and honey can be given as a drink regularly through the day. *Garlic perles* can be given, two each morning and night.

● Essence of *cinnamon*, which is available from chemists or herbal suppliers, can be very effective for persistent coughs and catarrh. Use $\frac{1}{2}$ teaspoon (2–3ml) in a little warm water three times daily.

● Essential oils can be used in baths, hand and foot baths, for inhalations, vaporizers, and chest massage. Choose from *eucalyptus*, *lavender*, *lemon*, *pine* and *thyme*.

Dietary Treatment of Coughs

If the cough accompanies a fever and the child is unwell, it is best to give no solid food and plenty to drink. Once the appetite returns and the fever is gone, give only light foods, no milk or meat, except chicken, plenty of fresh fruit, vegetables, vegetable soups and casseroles, vegetable and fruit juices and brown rice.

• A useful recipe to help ease bronchial congestion is to slice an onion into a small bowl and drizzle honey over it. Cover and leave to stand over-night. Spoon the liquid to the child, in acute infections every two hours and for chronic coughs two or three times a day.

• Fruit salads with grated ginger will help to shift residual catarrh. Pineapples, grapes, lemons, oranges and grapefruit will all help to loosen mucus.

• Stewed apples with plenty of cinnamon and cloves are also useful.

• Hot lemon and honey can be taken frequently to soothe irritation, and help to dispel mucus and resolve the infection.

• Blackcurrant tea is often very effective for sore throats, coughs and catarrh. You could also make blackcurrant syrup which could be added to other herbal teas you prepare, to sweeten the taste.

Blackcurrant Syrup

1 cupful blackcurrants (fresh or frozen)
$\frac{3}{4}$ pint (450ml) of water
$\frac{1}{2}$ cup runny honey
$\frac{1}{4}$ cup brown sugar

Pound the blackcurrants. Dissolve the honey and brown sugar in the water in a saucepan on the stove. Pour over the blackcurrants. Leave to cool. Strain. Take 1–2 tablespoons (20–40ml) every few hours. Store in the fridge and use within three days.

• Supplements of garlic perles, vitamin C and cod liver oil can be taken to help the immune system. In acute infections, one or two garlic perles and 100mg vitamin C (chewable for children) can be taken every two or three hours; in chronic conditions, give three times daily. In either instance 1 teaspoon (5ml) of cod liver oil can be taken daily.

If any cough does not respond to treatment within a few days; if there are any breathing difficulties; if there is any blueness around the mouth or if there is any fever over 102°F (38.8°C), which will not respond to treatment, call your doctor.

Raspberry Cough Syrup

This marvellous recipe is an old traditional remedy for coughs, including whooping cough. It tastes delicious and can be given on its own, or mixed with other teas or tinctures to make them more palatable. It is made in two stages.

First, cover $1\frac{1}{2}$lb (700g) fresh raspberries with 2 pints (1200ml) of cider vinegar. Leave for 24 hours. Press and strain. To each pint (600ml) of liquid, add 1lb (450g) of raw cane sugar. Boil and skim off. Cool.

Second, for each pint (600ml) of raspberry and cider vinegar mixture, take 1lb (450g) of honey. To each 1lb (450g) of honey, add 1 pint (600ml) water. Boil and skim. Cool.

Add the two liquids together with 1oz (25g) of *cloves* and $1\frac{1}{2}$ tablespoons (30ml) of *lobelia* tincture (if you cannot obtain *lobelia*, use *squills* or *thyme* instead). Leave to macerate and strain after two weeks. This will keep indefinitely.

WHOOPING COUGH

This begins with what appears to be a normal cold, which then develops into a cough. It involves infection by bacteria (*Bordatella pertussis*), which irritate the airways and cause them to become swollen and clogged by thick mucus. Gradually the coughing becomes more severe, with spasmodic coughing bouts, which can last up to a minute. These end with the characteristic 'whoop', as the child draws breath in, and the child may bring up some thick mucus and also vomit. If the coughing bout is prolonged, it can make breathing difficult. If it is not treated, the coughing phase can last over two months, during which time (and sometimes afterwards) there is risk of secondary infection (see Pneumonia, page 108 and Bronchitis, page 107), as it causes weakening of the chest, making it more susceptible to infection. After whooping cough, a child may 'whoop' when he next catches a cold or cough. This is simply the child repeating a habit learned during the coughing bouts, and not a return of the whooping cough.

Possible Symptoms of Whooping Cough

☐ Cold symptoms with a slight cough in the first week
Leading to
☐ Aches and pains
☐ Fever
☐ Cough, which increases, coming in short, sharp paroxysms
☐ Vomiting after a bout of coughing
☐ Coughing fits are worse at night and may cause sleeplessness
☐ In the third week, the child gets worse, and heavy spasms of coughing develop, often with the characteristic 'whoop'

Whooping cough can be a very worrying and distressing illness for both parents and children, and naturally it induces a lot of fear. It tends to be worse in small babies, who may not be so good at drawing the breath in over the swollen larynx (which causes the 'whoop') and are, therefore, more prone to breathing difficulties. However, the more reassuring aspect of whooping cough is that the onset is *gradual*. If there is whooping cough going around your neighbourhood and your child develops a cold and/or a cough, you can start herbal treatment immediately. You have from ten days to two weeks to treat the child, before the coughing becomes more serious, to prevent the whooping stage.

If you suspect that your child has whooping cough, you should contact your local practitioner for confirmation and advice. Do not send the child to school as it is a highly contagious disease.

Herbal Treatment of Whooping Cough

● At the first signs of a cold or slight cough, make a tea using the following prescription:

$\frac{1}{2}$ part *sundew* 1 part *coltsfoot* 1 part *elecampane* 1 part *squills* 1 part *thyme*.

Sweeten with *liquorice*, and add honey if necessary. Give the tea as often as you can, up to the equivalent of four to six cups a day.

Sundew This wonderful herb has been shown to be effective against a number of infecting organisms (streptococcus, staphylococcus and pneumococcus) as well as whooping cough. It contains a substance called plumbagin, which appears to be responsible for much of its beneficial effect. It also has a relaxing effect on the muscles in the bronchi, preventing them from going into spasms in a coughing bout. It is best used in small doses, and its effect has been confirmed to be most effective in whooping cough, especially when used with thyme.[1]

Squills This herb will help to liquefy the sticky mucus, making it easier to cough up and stopping it from blocking the airways. The soothing mucilage in the plant helps to relax the bronchial tubes, reducing the tendency to spasm.

Elecampane A specific for irritating coughs in children, this is particularly useful where there is profuse mucus as in whooping cough. It is relaxing to the bronchial muscles while, at the same time, stimulating the expulsion of mucus. It has an antibacterial action and is used effectively in bronchitis and pneumonia as well as whooping cough.

Coltsfoot Coltsfoot relaxes and soothes the chest, with a gently expectorant action, which helps to loosen and expel the mucus. It is a particularly good remedy for persistent coughs.

Thyme The volatile oils have an antiseptic action, which helps to resolve the infection. It is also a relaxant, reducing spasm in the chest while, at the same time, it is an expectorant, helping to loosen and expel the mucus. Thyme can be used for any cough with spasm, with other remedies or simply in thyme tea or syrup (see page 111), and whooping cough will, in most cases, respond to thyme when given on its own.

If they are treated properly when it first starts, the symptoms should not worsen to the point where the distressing coughing begins. If, however, you miss the first stage, and serious coughing sets in, you can still use the same recipe, giving tea every hour or so, and add one or two of the following herbs:

Wild Cherry Bark This has a powerful sedative action on the cough reflex, which is vital in the whooping stage.

Wild Lettuce A sedative and muscle relaxant, wild lettuce is especially useful where there is much fear and panic (it may be useful for parents as well). Tension will only aggravate the spasm in the bronchi, so it is most important that the child is kept as relaxed as possible.

Red Clover This herb helps to relax bronchial spasm while, at the same time, it helps expectoration of mucus.

Because it is so important to encourage your child to take the herbs, you will need to experiment to discover which is the best way to get him or her to take them in substantial amounts. You can give:

- ☐ Teas – to be taken as often as possible, sweetened with *liquorice*, *honey* or *aniseed*.
- ☐ Tinctures – easier because they are more concentrated. Between five and ten drops of the mixture can be given in *thyme syrup* or a drink every two hours. If the condition becomes more serious, they can be given every hour if necessary.
- ☐ Hand and foot baths – using teas or tinctures, diluted in water, two or four times daily.
- ☐ Inhalations or baths using strong infusions or tinctures in hot water.
- ☐ Essential oils – choose from *basil*, *cypress*, *eucalyptus*, *lavender*, *marjoram* or *thyme* and use them as inhalations, in vaporizers, in massage oils for the chest, feet or abdomen. A few drops can be put on the pillow at night, on a damp towel on the radiator or used in a plant spray to spray the room.
- ☐ Compresses – teas, tinctures or oils in warm water can be applied frequently to the chest.
- ☐ Choose three oils and put one drop of each into a little petroleum jelly and rub into the chest.

To Relax and Soothe the Chest

Garlic, with its antiseptic action in the chest is useful here and it also relaxes the muscle in the bronchial tubes and helps expectoration. It can be given in perles or juice, or in the following recipe.

Chop three heads of *garlic* and pour over ½ pint (300ml) of boiling water. Cover. Leave to macerate for a day. Strain. Give 1 tablespoon (20ml) every one or two hours. Use as a warm foot bath or chest compress also. Store in a refrigerator and use within three or four days.

Slippery elm food, made into a gruel and given three times daily, is also useful as it relaxes and soothes the chest, while being light, easy to digest and very nutritious.

Dietary Treatment of Whooping Cough

At the onset of cold or cough symptoms give only fruit or fruit and vegetables, with fruit juice, vegetable juice or herb teas sweetened with honey for a day or two. Then give only light food, with no milk, no sugar, no starchy foods, plenty of soups, grated vegetables, fresh fruit, chicken or fish.

Give supplements of cod liver oil (a teaspoon/5ml) daily, vitamin C (200mg three times daily) and *garlic* juice, honey or perles (every two hours).

General Advice for the Treatment of Whooping Cough

It is important that the child should rest as much as possible to give the body a chance to recuperate. You can give *camomile* tea to help the child to rest and sleep, and use stories, books or videos to encourage him or her to be quiet. Especially during a bad coughing phase, too much exertion can bring on coughing and deplete the child's energy, so it is best to find things to keep the child calm. Your child may need a lot of reassurance, especially during coughing fits, and may feel better if you hold him or her and talk to help stop panic, which will only make the breathlessness and coughing worse.

- During coughing, sit the child up, leaning forward, and encourage him or her to spit up the phlegm into a bowl.

- Bach flower remedies – *Rock Rose* for panic

or *Rescue Remedy* – can be used liberally for both parents and child.

• If your child vomits after coughing, once the coughing bout has stopped, make sure that he or she drinks plenty of herb teas sweetened with honey to keep the strength up and prevent dehydration.

• If the coughing becomes bad it may be best to sleep in the room with the child at night so that you can be there to offer reassurance and keep an eye on things. Coughing is very often worse at night than in the daytime.

• Make sure there is plenty of fresh air in the room, and keep chemicals and cigarette smoke well away.

• Once the whooping cough has gone, should there be another cough or difficulty breathing or should the child seem unwell, it may be that a secondary chest infection has set in. Consult your local practitioner for confirmation. If so, continue treatment along the same lines, until all symptoms are clear.

Call your doctor immediately if the baby or child is having breathing difficulties, if there is blueness around the mouth or if there is excessive vomiting which could lead to risk of dehydration.

Prevention of Whooping Cough

A child is more prone to whooping cough if he or she is generally run down and lacking in vitality, particularly if this is due to recurrent respiratory infections, with coughs, or there is a history of asthma or asthma occurs in the family.

A fairly robust child will probably throw whooping cough off fairly easily, but if there is a weakness in the chest and a tendency to chronic catarrh, or if there is weakness or congestion in the digestive tract, with a history of constipation, diarrhoea or tendency to tummy upsets, the child may be more susceptible to whooping cough, which could develop into the whooping stage unless properly treated.

It is important to iron out any weaknesses of the immune system, any tendencies to infection, catarrh or digestive disturbances as they arise so that your child is able to withstand infection, by whooping cough or anything else, as robustly as possible (see Immune System, page 61).

If there is whooping cough in your neighbourhood you can give teas of *agrimony, coltsfoot, elderflowers, elecampane* and *thyme* mixed in equal parts and sweetened with honey, three times daily. This will help to strengthen the chest and clear phlegm as well as any digestive congestion. Also give plenty of *garlic* and vitamin C.

ASTHMA

Asthma occurs when the bronchial tubes and bronchioles constrict, causing difficulty breathing, particularly when exhaling (breathing out), when a characteristic wheezing sound can be heard. It is a condition in which the child has asthma 'attacks', between which he or she is quite well. It is related to low general health, weak lungs, allergies and stress.

Causes of Asthma

An asthma attack may be triggered by a variety of different factors, which may act separately or in combination:

Allergy Many asthmatics are allergic to pollen, house dust, animal fur and a variety of foods, and may also be prone to other allergic reactions, such as eczema and hay fever. (For background causes of asthma see Allergies, page 67).

Symptoms of Asthma Attack

(An attack may last for a few minutes or a few hours.)

☐ Acute breathlessness
☐ Wheezing
☐ Difficulty breathing out
☐ Sneezing, itching of the nose may also occur
☐ Coughing

Irritation Asthma can be set off by a smoky or cold, foggy atmosphere. Certain household chemicals can also be culprits.

Infection Any respiratory infection (cough, cold or influenza, for example) can irritate the bronchial tubes and cause them to constrict.

Emotional factors These can play a part. Children with asthma may be being suffocated by an over-protective parent, or there may be nervousness, hypersensitivity, disharmony in the family or the surroundings, particularly insecurity, causing constriction in the chest. When asthma has been set off by something other, the anxiety that this may cause, and distress if the attack is severe, may aggravate it and make it worse.

Inherited Disposition A close relative may have asthma or eczema.

Digestive Disturbances These may irritate the vagus nerve, which feeds the stomach and the bronchial tubes, causing the constriction of muscles in the chest.

During an asthma attack, several factors combine to cause difficulty breathing: the muscles, arranged in rings in the bronchial tubes, tense up and narrow the airway; the mucous membrane lining the tubes swells and thickens, further narrowing the airway; and the mucous membrane secretes thick mucus, further filling the air space that remains.

If there are severe breathing difficulties, there may be a sense of suffocation and the child may panic; there may be blueness around the lips, indicating lack of oxygen. If this occurs, call the doctor immediately.

Between asthma attacks there can remain a chronic background wheeziness, which is worse on exertion, when running, playing or swimming, and during times of stress. It may vary from day to day, depending on the exposure to allergens and irritants. An asthmatic child may well have a tendency to chronic catarrh or repeated respiratory infections which weaken the lungs.

Asthma is not normally found in children under two years of age, although other respiratory disturbances cause wheezing, both in infants and older children: bronchiolitis in infants causes wheezing and trouble with breathing in and out when the bronchioles become inflamed and blocked (see page 108), and children with croup wheeze, but it is characterized by trouble breathing *in* and not *out* as in asthma (see page 116).

Asthmatic bronchitis affects children mostly between the ages of two and six. Wheezing is accompanied by a fever, dry cough and some difficulty breathing, and it is caused by constriction of bronchi and bronchioles, as a result of an allergic reaction to infection in the bronchi or to the mucus it produces. It normally occurs in children younger than those who normally develop classic asthma, but it tends to develop in allergic children and always occurs as a result of infection. Thus it requires treatment for the infection as well as the accompanying allergic response.

Prevention of Asthma

The most important line of treatment is to prevent attacks and, preferably, to resolve the chronic problem. This necessitates constitutional treatment of the child, and you will probably do best with professional advice, particularly if it is a serious case. It is important to attempt to discover which substances your child is allergic to or irritated by. Although he or she may react to a variety of things – foods, pollen, animal dander, feathers, plants, moulds or the house-dust mite, for example – it is an uphill struggle to prevent contact with these, and food is by far the easiest area to work with. If the culprit foods can be found and omitted from the diet, it takes a considerable strain off the debilitated immune system, which then has a greater ability to resist sensitivity to other substances such as animal dander or the house-dust mite, which are so much harder to avoid.

• The most common food allergens are milk produce, wheat, eggs, oranges and artificial colourings, flavourings and preservatives (particularly sulphur). If one of these foods, particularly milk, crops up again and again in your analysis of your child's diet, and the child has a particular liking for it, this is a good enough guide to which food to omit first. Do this for a month and, during this time, assess changes in the general vitality of the child, the condition of the chest and frequency of asthma attacks. If there is a significant change, stick to the same regime. If not, omit the next suspected food for a month and continue.

• While you embark on this voyage of discovery, you can treat the child with herbs, combining herbs to improve the function of the immune system and to decrease the allergic tendency, with herbs specifically to relax the bronchial tubes and expel the mucus. It is not enough simply to remove the offending allergic substances, even if the asthma improves, for the allergic tendency will remain, only to focus its attention later on some other food that is frequently eaten.

Herbal Treatment of Asthma

It may take a few months or even a year to treat asthma effectively, so it is important to be patient and not give up too easily. During this time, if your child already uses inhalers or other medication from the doctor, herbs can be used in conjunction with these. As the condition improves, you should find that you will need the inhalers or steroids less and less and that you can *gradually* withdraw them. This is best done with the help of a herbal practitioner.

• Herbs for the immune system, such as *borage*, *camomile*, *garlic*, *liquorice*, *wild yam* and *yarrow* can be combined with herbs to relax the bronchi and expel the mucus, such as *coltsfoot*, *grindelia*, *hyssop*, *lungwort*, *mullein*, *sundew* and *thyme*, and soothing herbs to relieve irritation in the chest; choose from *borage*, *comfrey*, *marshmallow*, *mullein* and *plantain*.

• *Liquorice* is a very interesting herb in this context. It has soothing, expectorant properties, and it helps to support the adrenal glands, providing a natural counterpart to cortisone and helping to reduce the effects of stress and allergic reactions, which is particularly useful for children using cortisone inhalers or internal medication, for which you wish to find an alternative.

• Herbs that support the nervous system, that help to relax the child and that counter stress and tension can be added if you think it appropriate for your child. Choose from *camomile*, *hops*, *limeflowers*, *skullcap* and *vervain*.

• For particular emotional difficulties that you feel are related to your child's asthma, it is well worth looking at the appropriate *Bach Flower Remedy* (see page 165). For an acute asthma attack Dr Bach's *Rock Rose* or *Rescue Remedy* can be given frequently, every few minutes if necessary, to relieve distress and panic.

• During an attack, hot foot baths can be made using the same herbs chosen for taking in infusions. Hot compresses of the same herbs can be applied frequently to the chest.

• A useful remedy for asthma, which may be used in these different ways, is to make an infusion of equal parts of *borage*, *camomile*, *coltsfoot*, *elecampane* and *thyme*. Add two parts of this infusion to one part *ginger* and *liquorice* decoction. Give ½ teaspoon (2–3ml) every 15–60 minutes, depending on how severe the attack is.

• *Thyme* tea alone is excellent for your children to strengthen the chest and relieve mild asthma.

• Because asthma is a serious condition, it is well worth visiting a medical herbalist, who will give you support and advice while you treat your child. There are several marvellous and famous herbs for asthma, such as *ephedra*, *lobelia* and *jimson weed*, which can be prescribed by a herbalist but are not freely available over the counter.

Dietary Treatment of Asthma

Give plenty of herbal teas to drink during an asthma attack, but give no food until the chest has settled down. The following foods are useful to counter the problem generally:

☐ Pure, unrefined sunflower seed oil, which contains inulin (which is effective for the treatment of asthma)

☐ Foods rich in vitamin A – carrots, spinach, peas, beetroot, fish liver oils, watercress, apricots

☐ Foods rich in calcium (see page 177)

☐ Garlic for the immune system

☐ Vitamin C containing foods to stimulate the expulsion of mucus from the chest and enhance the immune system

☐ Drinks of lemon and honey to help clear the mucus

☐ 1 teaspoon (5ml) of cider vinegar in a cup of warm water, sweetened with honey, can be taken regularly; during attacks this can be sipped regularly to help stop the wheezing

☐ Avoid dairy produce, excess wheat products, sugar and additives

General Advice in the Treatment of Asthma

Deep Breathing Asthma can be aggravated by faulty breathing. Practise deep breathing exercises regularly with your child to improve lung function as well as to help calm emotional stress – breathing has a direct connection to feelings and state of mind.

Abdominal breathing is easily learned and is simple to practise with your asthmatic child. As you slowly breathe in, your abdomen should expand outwards and, as you breathe out, it relaxes down again. If you use the abdomen instead of the top part of the lungs, your breathing will be more relaxed, and, if you count while you breathe, you will gain control over the breath. You can begin by breathing in for three seconds and out for three seconds. If the child finds this easy, gradually increase the time it takes to breathe in and out. Because the difficulty with asthmatics is with breathing out, shape the mouth as if to whistle and blow the breath out as slowly as possible.

Negative Ions Inhaling negative ions is very helpful to many asthma sufferers. These are released from running water, so being near rivers, waterfalls, the sea, or even the shower in the bathroom can be very therapeutic.

Avoidance of Colds Because coughs and colds often bring on an attack and, if frequent, can actually weaken the lungs and predispose to asthma developing in a child, they should be treated at their onset and preferably avoided (see Immune System, page 61).

Allergens Look carefully at your child's diet, and keep potential allergens – milk, wheat and eggs, for example – to a minimum. Restrict the use of sugar, avoid artificial additives and refined foods, and give plenty of fresh fruit and vegetables, nuts, seeds, grains (not so much wheat), beans and pulses.

If your child suffers from other allergies, it is important that they are treated constitutionally (see Allergies, page 67).

Fresh Air and Exercise Encourage your child to take plenty of fresh air and outdoor exercise. All exercise should be gentle; vigorous exercise, especially in cold air, can bring on an attack.

Relaxation Encourage plenty of rest and relaxation to allow the child's body to heal itself. Do not overstimulate the child and try to discourage frightening or over-exciting games or television programmes. Perhaps you could put time aside to play quiet games, or read to your child and engender quietness within. Meditation can be especially helpful. Emotional stresses and strains within the family may be better discussed openly so that any exaggerated fears may be dispelled and there is an opportunity for mutual support.

Herbal Teas If there is a history of asthma or allergies in the family, or if there is tendency to wheezing during respiratory infections or to frequent coughs and colds, give herbal teas regularly as a preventative. Mix equal parts of *camomile*, *coltsfoot*, *elecampane* and *thyme* and give hot infusions, sweetened with honey, two or three times daily.

Eczema Eczema, which is suppressed with the use of hydrocortisone cream, can frequently develop into asthma as the illness goes further into the body.

HAY FEVER

Strictly speaking, hay fever is an allergic reaction to grass pollen, which usually occurs at its worst in May, June and July. The term was originally related to symptoms caused by dust when hay-making, and it involves itching of the nose and eyes, sneezing, red, inflamed and watery eyes and runny nose, with clear discharge and sometimes wheezing. It can trigger an asthma attack in an asthmatic child. These symptoms can, however, occur at other times of the year in reaction to a variety of other substances, including pollens from trees and flowers and various foods, and they are often referred to as 'hay fever'. They are also known as allergic rhinitis or seasonal rhinitis. They are all related to an over-sensitivity of the mucous membranes in the respiratory tract.

True hay fever occurs once the pollen from grasses becomes airborne, and it is worse and often very tiresome during hot dry weather, when the pollen count in the atmosphere rises. It is worse near new-mown grass and when the hay is cut in the summertime. Rainy weather reduces the amount of pollen carried about in the air.

Hay fever rarely occurs before the age of five, and children tend to be worse affected during adolescence. Very often, these are children with an existing allergic tendency, who perhaps exchange a former allergic reaction, such as eczema, for hay fever (see Allergies, page 67).

General Treatment of Hay Fever

Like other allergies, hay fever is related to the immune system. There may be an inherited disposition to allergies and/or hay fever, or it may be that poor diet or low general health has made the immune system and respiratory tract over-susceptible to pollen. It often occurs in children who have a tendency to chronic catarrh or frequent respiratory infections, as the mucous membranes are already irritated. It appears that hay fever has become widespread only in the last 150 years or so, during which time the consumption of sugar has increased dramatically. It could be that the harmful effects that sugar has on the immune system are related to the increase in allergies that is clearly plaguing the Western world.

- Wheat is a member of the grass family. If wheat is removed from the diet during the hay fever season, the allergic symptoms can very often be dramaticaly reduced, if not completely eliminated. It appears that when the burden of wheat eaten in the diet is removed from the body, the body is better able to cope with the extra exposure to grass-related substances during the hay fever season. I have seen this work well countless times, and it is well worth the effort. It is also a good idea to cut out cow's milk produce, sugar and refined carbohydrates at the same time.

- There is a way of desensitizing a child before the hay fever season to prevent the allergic reaction to pollen. Honey, and especially the wax capping on honeycombs, contains pollen collected by the bees. For two to four months before the hay fever season, give a dessertspoonful or two (10–20ml) of honeycomb or honey with each meal. Local honey will contain the type of pollens in the surrounding countryside to which your child is likely to be exposed, so this is best. This preventative treatment often works very well.

- It is important to build up the immune system and to enhance general health for a few months before the hay fever season begins so that the system can cope with the high levels of pollen in the air when it comes. This can be done using herbs and diet for the immune system (see page 70). Choose from *borage*, *echinacea*, *garlic*, *ginseng*, *liquorice* and *wild yam*, and continue with your chosen herbs throughout the hay fever season.

Herbal Treatment of Hay Fever

The following herbal remedies can be given; they help to reduce hay fever symptoms as well as supporting the immune system. Choose from *camomile*, *echinacea*, *elderflowers*, *euphorbia*, *eyebright*, *marshmallow* and *wild yam*. These can be taken in hot infusion, three to six times daily depending on the severity of the hay fever.

Ephedra This herb is a specific for hay fever. It is one of the few herbs whose use is restricted, because it is toxic in large quantities, but it can be obtained through a herbal practitioner. My favourite prescription for hay fever is equal parts of *echinacea, ephedra, eyebright and euphorbia* given in tincture three to six times daily.

If your child's hay fever does not respond to any of the above, you should seek professional help.

● If the mucus is particularly persistent, *elderflower* and *ginger* tea and honey may well help to clear it. *Garlic*, either as juice, perles or honey, is helpful and should be taken every two hours if necessary.

● Steam inhalations of *camomile* – using strong tea or two drops of essential oil in a bowl of hot water – can be very helpful in reducing the allergic response and toning the mucous membranes. These can be given two or three times a day in conjunction with herbal teas.

● You should also continue with the honey or honeycomb throughout the hay fever season.

● Finally, because all allergic reactions, including hay fever, are related to a complex range of background causes and not only the offending allergens, it is always necessary to assess each individual child's constitution and lifestyle.

THE EYES

A child's eyes can tell you a lot about that child's health and happiness – whether they are bright or sparkling, dull and half-closed, or shifty with tension or anxiety. The expression in the eyes is one of the ways in which a parent first tells if their child is off-colour or unhappy.

Eyes have other functions. They are responsible for connecting us to light – life-giving sunlight – which is responsible not only for our vision but also influences our physical and mental well-being. Sunlight affects the secretion of endorphins, hormone-like substances that give us a feeling of well-being. During the winter months in the Northern hemisphere the many hours of darkness mean that many who do not get adequate sunlight suffer from a kind of depression, known as seasonal affective disorder (SAD), and a reduced resistance to infection, so it is important to encourage your children to spend time playing or walking outside in the fresh air and sunlight, even on a dull day in the winter.

Crying and the production of tears is another important function of the eyes. Tear drops produced when we cry contain endorphins, opiate-like substances, which actually calm us down. It may be that we should not be too ready to stop a child from crying when he or she needs to – not only can it release pent-up emotions but can also prove to be therapeutically calming. In addition, tears are constantly washed in tiny amounts across the eyes to protect the eye from damage and to clear away any debris in the eye.

The eyelids also protect the eyes. Their inner surfaces and the visible surface of each eye are covered with a delicate protective membrane known as the conjunctiva. Tears produced by tear glands lubricate the conjunctiva and drain into the channels passing into the nose. The eyelids and conjunctiva are prone to various problems which can be successfully treated using herbs.

CONJUNCTIVITIS

This is an inflamed condition of the conjunctiva, which can be caused by an infection, injury to the eye from dirt, dust or pollution, a foreign body stuck in the eye or an allergy. The white of the eyes becomes pink or red, and can feel sore and irritated and aggravated by bright lights. The eyes may be weepy, and a discharge may cause crusting and glueing up of the eyes and eyelashes in the morning after sleep. If your child is prone to repeated attacks or chronic conjunctivitis it may be caused by irritation from chemicals in the environment or by food allergy, often to dairy produce or candida (see pages 67 and 73). Conjunctivitis also often accompanies hay fever.

BLEPHARITIS

This is inflammation of the eyelids, which is most often due to infection or allergy. The eyelids are red and a little swollen, and they can feel irritated or sore. There may be a pus-like discharge causing sticking of the eyes and lashes after sleep, as in conjunctivitis.

Herbal Treatment of Conjunctivitis and Blepharitis

Both conjunctivitis and blepharitis are treated similarly.

• Bathe the eyes three times a day with an infusion prepared from previously boiled or distilled water, or a decoction of *camomile, chickweed, comfrey, elderflowers, eyebright, golden seal, marigold, marshmallow, plantain, raspberry leaves* or *rosemary*.

• A very effective combination of *camomile, eyebright* and *marigold* is one of my favourite recipes for sore, inflamed eyes, but any of the above herbs may be used singly or in combinations.

• Tea bags of any of these can be soaked in boiling water and taken out when luke warm. You can place them over the eye for 5–10 minutes – Use a different tea bag for each eye so as not to spread the infection.

• Distilled *witch hazel* or *rose water* can also be very beneficial. These can be combined with herbal infusions or decoctions or tinctures. For example, mix 10 drops of *eyebright* in 3 tablespoons (55ml) of *rose water*. Always make sure that you sterilize the eye bath before you use it for children who are old enough to manage it. For younger children, use cotton wool – separate pieces for each eye – to wipe the eyes from the outer part of the eye towards the nose.

• It is always best to treat the child internally at the same time to enhance the immune system's ability to deal with either infection, inflammation or allergy, and to treat the eyes specifically. Give teas of *camomile, cleavers, echinacea, elderflowers, eyebright* or *hyssop* three times daily, singly or in combination. Always make sure that *eyebright* forms part of your mixture. Sweeten with honey or fruit juice if you wish.

• If your child has repeated attacks of conjunctivitis or blepharitis and you suspect an allergic reaction, it is important to isolate the allergen and remove it as far as possible. Use *camomile* to bathe the eyes, and *camomile, yarrow* or *lemon balm* given internally three times a day.

• Give plenty of foods containing vitamins C, A and B and supplements of vitamin C and garlic.

• See also Allergies (page 67), Candidiasis (page 73), Hay Fever (page 120) and Treatment of Infections (page 72).

STYES

An inflammation of a hair follicle of an eyelash can cause a pus-filled swelling on the eyelid, usually on the lower one. A stye can feel sore and swollen, and it generally comes to head and bursts within four or five days. A stye is usually a sign that a child is tired or run down and will be encouraged by rubbing or touching the eyes frequently and pulling eyelashes. It can be associated with a more general irritation of the eyelids or with blepharitis. Try to discourage your child from touching the affected eye, as this can cause a stye in the other eye.

Treatment of Styes

If the stye is painful, apply a warm compress for a few minutes every two or three hours to soothe the discomfort and to help bring the stye to a head. Use an infusion or decoction of *burdock, camomile, elderflowers, eyebright, golden seal, marigold, marshmallow* or *plantain*. You can also use 5 drops of tincture in ½ cup of distilled water, mixed with *rose water* or *witch hazel*.

• Give teas internally to help de-toxify the system and increase resistance. Make tea from *burdock, echinacea, eyebright* and *red clover*, and give it, with a little *liquorice*, three times daily. *Garlic* and vitamin C supplements are also recommended.

THE NERVOUS SYSTEM

The whole person is made up not only of the physical body, but also of the emotions, the mind and the spirit. Just as disorders of the physical body can affect the way we think and feel, so every thought and emotion has a direct effect on the physical body. Disharmony and negativity in our thoughts and feelings can diminish energy and vitality and reduce resistance, and are expressed as disease in the body; harmonious thoughts and feelings, such as hope, faith, love and happiness, create corresponding physical well-being, affecting as they do the chemical composition of the tissues and secretions of the body in a positive way.

A study of the nervous system clearly illustrates the relationship between mind and body. The nervous system is part of our physical body, it is made up of nerve cells (neurones) and fibres, which comprise the brain and spinal cord, the peripheral nerves and the autonomic nervous system. Yet it expresses thoughts and emotions as well as controlling physical activities and sensations . . . there is really very little separation between mind and body except that which we have created. Disease in the physical nervous system will create psychological imbalances, and negative emotions can create physiological illness. This disharmony in the body can be treated through a psychological approach – counselling or psychotherapy, for instance – and disharmony in the mind can be treated through a healing of the nervous system as a tissue, through herbs and diet. Using herbal medicines and healthy eating, the nervous system can be fed and strengthened, its health enhanced and its function improved and, in this way, the behaviour of a 'difficult' or unhappy child may radically change.

This connection between mind and body should underline that, when we care for our children, we do not simply have to look after their bodily needs – diet and lifestyle, fresh air, exercise and so on. We are also responsible for nurturing, with love, stability and harmony, a healthy mind and emotions, for instilling in them creative, positive thoughts and feelings, and for allowing the free flow of their imagination and intuition. At the same time, we need to understand and support them through the difficult times and negative reactions they may have as they journey through childhood. It is a learning experience for all of us.

BEHAVIOURAL PROBLEMS

All children can be difficult at times and some children cause extreme anxiety and despair to their parents because of their over-frequent disruptive or difficult behaviour. They seem to be at odds with themselves and the people around them, and this can be very exhausting. Some children are over-aggressive; others have frequent temper tantrums about apparently insignificant events; others hold their breath in fits of rage and are unable to let go, going red and purple in the face until they nearly pass out; others refuse to go to sleep, either at night or in the day, except in short bursts. Naturally, there are numerous causes of such problems, which can originate on both physical and emotional levels.

Physical Causes

Almost any kind of physical imbalance can affect a child's behaviour; this becomes clear during acute infections when a child may cry or cling a lot.

Digestive Imbalance When we consider long-term behavioural problems, we may look for a low-grade, chronic imbalance – digestive or bowel problems, for example. Loose, smelly stools may indicate a malabsorption problem, depleting the child nutritionally and creating poor health. Constipation will lead to the accumulation of toxins in the body and will affect the mind, producing lethargy and irritability and sometimes pretty poisonous behaviour! Liver congestion from over-eating, from junk food or from foods full of artificial additives or heavy metals will affect the way a child feels, from being irritable and angry to being lethargic and depressed. It is certainly worth getting a complete physical check-up for any difficult child.

Food Allergy One major cause of difficult behaviour in children is food intolerance or allergy. Many parents will be familiar with the effect of chocolate on children; you may notice that your child always comes home from a birthday party, where chocolate and junk foods abound, in a foul mood. Cola drinks, sugar and food colouring and additives (particularly tartrazine) can all have devastating effects on a child. Another common allergy is to milk produce, which can cause a variety of emotional disturbances, ranging from insomnia to temper tantrums, aggression and black moods. Gluten and corn may also be culprits. Allergic reactions to foods can be mild or very extreme. Sometimes they can primarily affect the tissues of the brain, causing what is known as a cerebral allergy and sometimes resulting in psychotic behaviour. If you observe that your child easily becomes lethargic, irritable, depressed or difficult, and immediately feels better after eating a certain food, such as sugar, chocolate or milk, this could point to the allergic food, or it could indicate low blood sugar (hypoglycaemia, see below). It is obviously best omitted from the diet for a good period of time while the allergy is treated.

Nutritional Deficiencies Nutritional deficiencies can also disrupt the normal function of the nervous system. These can be easily created by a diet that is high in sugar and refined foods and low in vegetables and fruit and unrefined oils. Such diets tend to be lacking in B complex vitamins, vitamins C and E, and a wide range of minerals and trace elements, including calcium, magnesium, zinc and manganese, all of which are vital to normal brain function. These nutritional deficiencies can be the cause of food allergies as well.

Low Blood Sugar Low blood sugar can also cause mood swings and erratic behaviour. This will be evident when a child is moody and irritable, pale or dark round the eyes until a meal, after which the former sunny character will emerge again. A major cause of low blood sugar is the over-consumption of sugar and refined carbohydrates – in cakes, biscuits and sweets – which places a strain on the pancreas and liver. It often occurs in allergic children. It can be easily put right by a low sugar, wholefood diet. If it does not respond, consult your practitioner.

Hyperactivity If there is restlessness, over-activity, sleeplessness, tantrums and disruptive behaviour, your child may be hyperactive (see page 126).

Worms Worms, which disturb normal bowel functions, can cause irritability and moodiness, lethargy and poor sleep (see page 140).

Heavy Metals Heavy metal toxicity – lead from car fumes if you live on a busy road, for instance – can affect behaviour. If you suspect this, a hair test would determine the matter.

In addition, lack of fresh air and exercise, over-exposure to polluted smoky atmospheres and too much television can all create problems.

The treatment of the physical causes will depend on the nature of specific imbalances in each child. You may need to consult your local herbal practitioner if you do not feel clear about your direction here.

Emotional Causes

Birth Trauma Emotional problems can go as far back as the birth of the child. If the birth was long, difficult or traumatic, oxygen was short or drugs were used, these could all affect the baby. *Bach Flower Remedies* can be very useful here, even if the birth was several years ago. The passage through the birth canal can affect the central nervous system, and this is best detected by a cranial osteopath, who can often work wonders if the child has been difficult since birth.

Family Problems It may be that a 'difficult' child is simply reflecting what is going on within the family unit. Children are very intuitive and can pick up whatever tensions are flying about – anxieties of either parent, strife between partners, grief or fear – and they may react without knowing why. Sometimes children feel responsible for emotional difficulties experienced by their parents. If there are particular difficulties within the family, it is important to make a special effort to be extra-caring and nurturing to a possibly insecure child.

Life Changes There are certain changes in life that each child has to go through but that may prove difficult for some. The transition from being an only child to being the older brother or sister may be one of the hardest. If your young child is being aggressive – biting, kicking younger children, taking their toys and making it impossible for people to want to play with him or her – it may well be that he or she is hitting out, because he or she really wants to hit the new-born baby but knows that is not allowed. Taking toys or disrupting games may mean that the child wants to get back at someone or that toys represent love and the child feels that he or she is not getting enough and is jealous of other children who are. Other difficult periods may be connected with starting at play school, or moving house or school, realizing that homework is here to stay or moving into adolescence.

Treatment

There may be several ways you can help to ease your child through the changes. The best you can do is to be there and be supportive.

• The *Bach Flower Remedies* (page 165) are wonderfully effective in many cases; choose three or four from the list that suit your child and vary the prescription when you need to. You may need to continue with the remedies in this way over several weeks or even months.

• Make sure that you are providing your child with all that the nervous system needs to be able to function normally through diet. Vitamins B, C and E, calcium, magnesium, manganese and zinc to name a few, are all vital. During times of emotional difficulties the body will metabolize these nutrients far faster than normal, so supplements may be necessary. A multi-mineral and vitamin tablet, with extra vitamin C tablets and plenty of fruit and vegetables, nuts and seeds and unrefined oils in the diet, with no junk food and very little sugar, would be helpful.

• Herbal remedies can be used to support a stressed or run-down nervous system, helping it to cope better with what life is presenting. *Vervain* and *skullcap* are wonderfully balancing and strengthening. These can be taken as teas or tinctures three times daily.

• Oats are food for the nervous system. They act as a very beneficial tonic and can be taken in a decoction or tincture of *wild oats* three times daily, or in food as porridge, muesli, flapjacks and so on.

• For very tense and anxious children, *camomile*, *limeflower* and *skullcap* will prove helpful.

• Tonics for the adrenal glands, which are always overworked in these conditions, can be combined in your prescription. *Borage* and *liquorice* can be useful.

• Liver remedies will help a sluggish or over-worked liver or an erratic pancreas where there is low blood sugar, allergy or heavy metal toxicity, and they may prove very helpful where there is anger, irritability or depression. *Dandelion root* and *rosemary* can be combined with *peppermint* to soften the blow of the bitter herbs to the taste buds.

• Dilute essential *oils of lavender* and *camomile* can be used for baths, massages and inhalations. Children love to be massaged – it feels wonderful, and is very soothing and comforting to a tense, insecure or frightened child.

• Several physical conditions have a particularly strong relationship to the state of the nervous system:

☐ Allergies – asthma, hay fever, eczema
☐ Irritable coughs
☐ Bowel problems – constipation, diarrhoea, wind
☐ Stomach upsets, tummy aches, nausea
☐ Lowered resistance to infections, producing recurrent illness

If you feel that stress plays a part in any of these problems, you can support the nervous system and add the above tonics to other prescriptions you may be using. In many ways, a certain degree of stress can actually be of benefit, as it can accelerate learning at school, and adrenalin may improve performance during exams. However, even if the 'stress' seems positive to you, if it is prolonged it can be exhausting and debilitating to the child, so it is still worth supporting the child with nervine herbs and healthy eating.

There are other ways of helping a child to deal with stress when it becomes a problem:

☐ Breathing exercises
☐ Relaxation exercises
☐ Physical exercise – gym, games, martial arts, yoga
☐ Music and relaxation tapes are useful; you can listen to them with your child and you will both benefit
☐ Do creative or constructive and positive things together and try to capture the child's imagination – painting, crafts, singing, making up poems, for example; singing is of particular interest, as it helps

with control of breath and encourages correct abdominal breathing, which is very calming. Try repetitive chants together – many children love them

Any of the measures you choose to use for your child are certainly beneficial for parents of difficult children, who naturally may become worn out and frazzled, weepy or despairing, especially when there are long-term sleeping problems, meaning that parents are chronically exhausted. They, too, can use the herbal tonics, and should find them very restoring.

HYPERACTIVITY

If your child is very demanding, cries easily, has a poor attention span, is very excitable, extremely restless, has little apparent need of sleep and exhibits aggressive or disruptive behaviour, it may well be that he or she is hyperactive. Boys with blond hair and blue eyes are apparently more than normally prone.[2] Hyperactive children may also be dyslexic.

Sometimes, hyperactivity can be hard to diagnose, as it varies in degree from one child to another. It could simply be that your child is very intelligent, easily bored and needs a lot of stimulation.

Causes of Hyperactivity

• Hyperactivity is often related to food intolerance, particularly to certain food colourings (including those given in orthodox medicines for children, such as Calpol), flavourings, dairy produce, salicylates, wheat or gluten, chocolate, caffeine in cola drinks, eggs and citrus fruits, especially oranges. There is often a history of allergies, such as asthma, eczema, hay fever or migraine, in the family.

• Pollution can have some effect. Inhaling or ingesting toxic metals, such as lead, cadmium and aluminium, may affect brain function, as may organic solvents in, for example, felt-tip pens, cleaning fluids and aerosol sprays.

• Nutritional deficiencies, of, for example, iron, zinc, B vitamins, magnesium, resulting from a diet with insufficient fresh fruit and vegetables, whole grains and essential fatty

---

Symptoms of Allergies in the Hyperactive Child

A variety of physical symptoms may accompany behavioural problems in the hyperactive child, and these will be pointers towards nutritional deficiency and/or food allergy. They include:

☐ Dry skin, cradle cap or dandruff, dry cracked lips
☐ A family history of allergies
☐ Asthma, hay fever, eczema or other skin rashes
☐ Bed-wetting
☐ Frequent headaches
☐ Aching legs
☐ Fussy eating or poor appetite
☐ Excess dribbling, sweating or thirst
☐ Frequent infections & low resistance
☐ Catarrh
☐ Cravings for sweet foods
☐ Bloating 'wind' diarrhoea or constipation

---

acids, and aggravated by too much sugar and refined foods, are quite common, and can affect brain function, making it more susceptible to the adverse effects of toxic metals.

• Emotional upsets can contribute to hyperactivity by putting further stress on the nervous system and by increasing the body's metabolism of vital nutrients, thus increasing the risk of vitamin, mineral and trace element deficiencies.

• The consumption of alcohol, smoking and toxaemia during pregnancy, birth difficulties or ante-natal lack of oxygen can also result in hyperactivity.

• Candida albicans (thrush) infestation can occur due to overprescription of antibiotics or nutritional deficiencies, particularly of iron and zinc. If your child does not respond to the avoidance of possibly allergic food and dietary supplements, candida could be the problem (see page 73).

• Research suggests that passive smoking (breathing in the air in a room of smokers) is responsible not only for much respiratory illness in children, but also for increases in the incidence of allergy, intellectual problems and hyperactivity.

General Treatment of Hyperactivity

Suspected foods should be eliminated from the diet for an initial period of at least a month. If you find it hard to know where to begin, look at the list of possibly implicated foods and observe how much they crop up in your child's diet. Those that occur most frequently or that the child craves are the ones to omit first.

If you suspect that your child has an allergy, follow the treatment for Allergies (page 74).

• While investigating possible dietary causes, give supplements of necessary vitamins and minerals, including: a multi-mineral and vitamin tablet, zinc tablets (10mg daily), vitamin C tablets (500mg daily) and *evening primrose* oil (500mg capsule daily). These will help, not only to correct nutritional deficiencies but also to promote the excretion of toxic metals.

• Make sure that your child has regular meals and does not skip any. It is worth checking how much a fussy eater has during school meals, as some difficult behaviour can be caused by low blood sugar, resulting from infrequent meals.

• If you suspect candida, follow the advice on page 74.

• If there is no improvement after three or four weeks, seek advice from your local practitioner. It may be that there is another underlying illness that is related to the hyperactivity.

Herbal Treatment of Hyperactivity

Certain herbs help to cleanse the system of heavy metals. These include: *red clover*, *kelp* and *nettles* and they can be combined with tonic herbs for the nervous system, to support the nerves and the adrenal glands, which will be depleted from the constant overactivity. Tonics to the nervous system include *skullcap*, *vervain* and *wild oats*, while *borage* and *liquorice* will support the adrenal glands.

• See also herbs in general treatment of behavioural problems, page 125.

• To help your child sleep you may need herbs that are more relaxing: *camomile*, *catnip*, *cowslip*, *hops* and *limeflowers* can be given singly or together as tea before bed and again during the night should the child awake. They can also be added in strong infusions to bath water before bed (see also Insomnia, page 127).

INSOMNIA/SLEEPLESSNESS

On the whole, children need more sleep than adults, and they tend to sleep for at least twelve hours a night. However, many parents of young children have never had a full night's sleep since the child was born. In this case it is not only the child who needs treatment, but also the exhausted parents!

Causes of Insomnia

There are many different causes of sleep disturbance:

• The hyperactive child will have great difficulty getting off to sleep and will sleep for only a few hours at a time.

• The allergic child, with food intolerances, may have difficulty getting off to sleep or suffer a disturbed night, possibly with bad dreams.

• Nutritional deficiencies of, for example, zinc, manganese, vitamins C and B can contribute.

• *Candida albicans* (see page 73) can also be responsible.

• Stresses within the family or at school and insecurity from major changes (such as the arrival of a new baby, house or school move) can be important factors. Watching too much TV or a frightening bedtime story may excite or worry the child, who can be scared of the dark or of being alone in his bedroom. Nightmares related to this may wake the child.

• Getting overtired; one needs energy to sleep and relax.

- Lack of fresh air and exercise may contribute.

- Chronic problems, such as skin rashes, digestive problems, asthma or catarrh causing difficulty breathing, may disturb sleep.

- Acute infections, coughs, colds, fevers, headaches, will cause disturbed nights (see Fevers, Coughs and Colds, page 89).

General Treatment of Insomnia

First, it is important to ascertain the cause of your child's sleep problems. If there are other signs of hyperactivity (see page 126) or food allergy (see Immune System, page 67), explore those avenues and treat accordingly.

- Make sure your child is eating well, with plenty of whole foods and fruit, vegetables, nuts and seeds.

- Omit junk foods, especially sugar, from the diet and any stimulating or sugary drinks such as cocoa, chocolate, cola drinks, fizzy pop, tea or coffee, because toxins can affect the brain and nervous system, leading to poor sleep and nightmares.

- Hot drinks of yeast extract will help to boost the B vitamins in the body, and pure fruit juices will increase vitamin C, both of which are needed by the nervous system to ensure proper relaxation.

- Avoid eating just before bedtime.

- Foods containing plenty of calcium, such as parsley, watercress, dried figs, sesame seeds and tahini, will help to relax a child who is tense.

- A zinc supplement of 15mg, sucked as a lozenge, should be taken, as well as a children's multi-mineral and vitamin supplement, until a proper sleep pattern is well established.

Herbal Treatment of Insomnia

A warm bath at night before bed will help to relax the child, but make sure you don't allow the child to get too excited at bath time with games. A few drops of dilute oils of *camomile*, *clary sage* or *lavender* can be added to the bath water, or you could use strong infusions of *camomile*, *catnip*, *lavender*, *lemon balm* or *limeflowers*.

- Massage, using dilute oils of *camomile*, *lavender*, *neroli* or *rose* just before sleep, can be wonderfully soothing and reassuring for the child and induce sleep. It is a lovely way to treat your child, and allows time for some special moments together at the end of the day. Massage wherever your child likes best – it could be the feet, hands, tummy, back, neck or face.

- A cup of warm tea can be given before bed, and again in the night if the child awakes. Choose from *camomile*, *catnip*, *cowslip flowers*, *lemon balm* or *limeflowers* and sweeten with honey and flavour with *liquorice* if you wish.

Cowslip Syrup

You could also use cowslip syrup to soothe nerves and induce sleep. Pour a cup of boiling water over a handful of dried flowers. Add $\frac{1}{2}$ cupful of honey and leave to cool. Strain and bottle. Give 1–2 teaspoons (5–10ml) at night.

Herb pillows can be used to continue the herbal treatment through the night. These can be bought in some health food shops but you can easily make your own with dried herbs. They can be used singly or in combinations, which you can put together to make a pleasant-smelling blend. Try one yourself, too. Suitable herbs include *camomile*, *catnip*, *hops*, *lavender*, *lemon balm*, *limeflowers*, *orange blossom* and *sweet woodruff*.

- If your child wakes distressed, for example from a nightmare, always go straight to him or her and put the light on, and hold him or her close until the child is relaxed enough to go back to sleep.

- Never use bed as a punishment, as sleep could become associated with punishment.

- If you feel that your child is sleeping badly because of stress or emotional problems or is being disturbed by nightmares, you may need to treat the child in the daytime to help him to cope better with the emotional load and to relax any accumulating tension. *Camomile* and *lime-flower* tea can be combined with *skullcap* and taken three times daily. *Wild oats* can be taken in decoction once daily in the morning.

• *Catnip* as a tea, or in the bath, or a sleep pillow, is particularly recommended, for this is a tranquilizing herb, which is especially useful for allaying anxiety and fear from bad dreams and soothing nervousness to induce a restful sleep. Gypsies use a sprig of *rosemary* against nightmares; in Greece they use *basil*, and the Moroccans use sprigs of *southernwood*.

• The *Bach Flower Remedies* come into their own here. Choose the most appropriate for your child's needs and give them regularly through the day as well as before bed. *Aspen* and *Rescue Remedy* are particularly good for nightmares.

Treatment for the Parents

If you are feeling particularly tired, tinctures or teas of *wild oats*, *vervain* and *skullcap* can be taken three times a day. If your child's bad sleep pattern has resulted in a similarly poor sleep pattern in yourself, try a sleeping mix made from any of the herbs mentioned. Should you need something a little stronger, add one or two of the following: *cramp bark*, *pasque flower*,

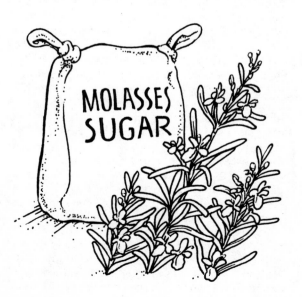

passionflower, *skullcap* and *valerian*, and take a strong infusion before bed, or 2–3 teaspoons (10–15ml) of tincture in a little warm water. Repeat if you wake up.

• Take a multi-mineral and vitamin tablet until you feel better, and make sure that you have plenty of C and B vitamins in your diet, as well as calcium and magnesium. Take 500mg vitamin C at night to help sleep. Cider vinegar and honey is also helpful taken at night. Never go to bed on a full stomach and avoid caffeinated drinks.

Rosemary Conserve

Rosemary is a wonderful herb for lifting the spirits when feeling tired and low. Rosemary conserve is an old-fashioned remedy, which provides a pleasant way to take the herb.

> $1\frac{1}{2}$ cups of molasses sugar
> $\frac{1}{2}$ cup of fresh flowering tips

Put in blender with a little infusion of rosemary to make it the consistency of honey. Pour into a jar with a stopper or tight-fitting lid. Store in a cold place or in a refrigerator. Take 1 teaspoonful 2–3 times daily over a few weeks. Continue for 3 weeks and no longer. This is also useful for headaches and colds and digestive upsets.

THE DIGESTIVE SYSTEM

The digestive system is vital for the conversion of the natural resources from the world around us into energy for our daily activities and for all the minute biochemical reactions within us. This conversion is essential to every living being, but particularly so for children, who are not only very active but whose bodies use nutrients at a faster rate than adults so that they can grow and develop.

The digestive tract runs for about 36 feet (11 metres) from the mouth to the anus. It is a hollow tube, which functions as a factory, processing food and producing energy to keep us alive and healthy. Because it opens at both ends to the outside world, and yet travels right through the middle of us, it means that there is constant interaction between our inner and outer environments. Some say we are what we

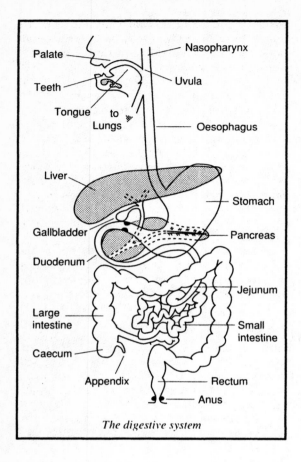

Palate

Teeth

Tongue
to
Lungs

Nasopharynx

Uvula

Oesophagus

Liver

Stomach

Gallbladder

Pancreas

Duodenum

Jejunum

Large
intestine

Small
intestine

Caecum

Appendix

Rectum

Anus

The digestive system

eat; others say we are what we absorb or assimilate. Whatever the truth, our health largely depends on how well our digestion makes the vital nutrients from our food available to us. The digestive tract is lined with a mucous membrane, which not only protects it but also serves to secrete digestive juices containing enzymes that are designed to break down food into a form we can absorb. Other digestive enzymes are supplied to the digestive tract by the liver, gall-bladder and pancreas.

The process of digestion begins in the mouth, where food is partly broken down by chewing and mixing with saliva, which contains digestive enzymes. It then passes down the oesophagus into the stomach, where it is broken down further by digestive juices, including hydrochloric acid. After this, the food moves into the small intestine, where it is mixed with more digestive enzymes, and bile from the gall-bladder and where most of the nutrients are absorbed into the bloodstream

and carried to the liver. The rest of the undigested food passes to the large intestine. Here, much of the water and some nutrients – such as sodium – are absorbed into the body, and the remainder passes to the rectum where it waits for evacuation.

Not only does this food conversion in the digestive tract *provide* energy but it also *requires* energy to carry out all the essential biochemical reactions involved in the process. If the digestive energy is weak or upset, problems arise, which not only produce symptoms directly relating to the digestive tract, such as stomach aches, diarrhoea or constipation, but also those affecting general health and energy, such as lethargy, irritability, inability to concentrate and disturbed sleep. It can cause nutritional deficiencies and often allergies.

The health of the digestive tract depends on several factors. First, regular peristaltic movements require sufficient roughage or fibre in the diet to pass food down the alimentary canal. Not only do we need to evacuate the food residues, but also the waste products of metabolism must be eliminated. If they are not, a toxic state of the bowel develops, which is prone to infection and the spread of toxins into the rest of the body. The condition of the bowels can fundamentally affect our general health and give rise to a wide variety of problems.

The autonomic nervous system regulates the circulation to and from the digestive tract, as well as the secretion of digestive juices. Stress can disrupt the digestion – for example, it can cause excess hydrochloric acid in the stomach, which can irritate and inflame and, in some adults, ulcerate the lining of the stomach or intestine. Absorption of food depends upon its being broken down by digestive juices, and this will vary from person to person – two people eating the same diet will end up with completely different amounts of nutrients. There is constant interaction between the brain and the digestive tract, making the process of digestion very susceptible to the effect of mind and emotion, personality and constitution. Often a child's stomach ache can be a straightforward reaction to an upset at home or at school or to too much excitement.

The right diet is vital to the health and normal function of the digestive tract. Over-refined foods, excess sugar, fizzy drinks, ice creams and fried foods can all irritate and create disturbances.

ACUTE STOMACH ACHES

Most children get stomach aches from time to time. They are often the result of eating the wrong foods, stress or excitement. They can also be due to food allergies and, of course to more serious problems, such as appendicitis, which requires prompt attention. Never feed a child who has stomach ache or any accompanying symptoms such as diarrhoea or vomiting. Give plenty to drink, and re-introduce light foods, such as vegetable soups, fruit purées and brown rice, once the symptoms have gone and before returning to normal eating.

Acute stomach ache can be related to any of the following: upset stomach, gastro-enteritis, vomiting, diarrhoea, food poisoning and dysentery, and to hiccups, stress and travel sickness.

UPSET STOMACH

Excitement, upset or over-eating the wrong foods (chocolate, sweets, fizzy drinks for example) or excess fruit in season (such as plums or sour apples) can cause tummy aches and sometimes vomiting or diarrhoea, but these will be easily resolved.

Treatment of Upset Stomach

• The best remedy is to give plenty to drink but no solid food until the child feels better, and encourage the child to rest.

• *Camomile*, *lemon balm* and *peppermint* can be given frequently as teas. These are excellent remedies to settle the stomach and calm the child.

• If the symptoms persist, call your practitioner.

GASTRO-ENTERITIS

This can occur commonly in children and will produce a tummy ache. It normally results from a viral infection in the digestive tract, which causes inflammation. In a natural response, the digestive tract tries to rid itself of the irritant through diarrhoea, vomiting or both. Normally this lasts for about twenty-four hours, by which time it is resolved. Should it last longer or cause severe symptoms, such as high fever and malaise or recurrent vomiting, call your practitioner.

Treatment of Gastro-enteritis

• If there is frequent vomiting or diarrhoea, especially in a baby or toddler, there is risk of dehydration (see page 135), so it is always important to give plenty to drink, either as herbal teas, dilute fruit or vegetable juices or as mineral water (and not milk).

• To help prevent dehydration and loss of electrolytes, give water with a pinch of salt and 1 teaspoon (5ml) of glucose per glassful, every 10–15 minutes.

• Spanish tummy or traveller's diarrhoea very often occurs when travelling abroad as the digestive tract struggles with new foods and new bacteria. *Garlic*, taken daily, will help to prevent tummy upset, as will fresh lemon juice taken before eating.

VOMITING

The ease with which children vomit depends, to a certain extent, on their age. Babies vomit easily, either because they have been overfed; they have too much wind; their stomachs are weak; their food has not agreed with them; or they have an infection (see Treatment for Babies, page 50).

Toddlers vomit if they have over-eaten or have eaten badly, something that has not agreed with them – that is, they have a tummy upset or an allergic reaction; they have an infection, they have a weak stomach, they have got upset or over-excited; or they have, or have had, a cold or cough with much phlegm, which has been swallowed and accumulated in the stomach.

Treatment of Vomiting

Overeating

If a child has over-eaten or reacted badly to a

type of food there is vomiting of largely undigested food. In a baby this can be immediately after a feed; in an older child it could be several hours later and typically at night. There is usually a stomach ache and nausea, which builds up gradually to vomiting. The child is often upset and weepy, and will need comfort and reassurance, especially if it happens at night.

You can give herbal teas, taken slowly in sips so that they do not come straight back again, made from any of the following, either singly or in combination: *camomile*, *fennel*, *lemon balm* or *peppermint*. These can also be given in tincture form, 5–10 drops in a glass of water.

Infection

If the child has an infection, the vomiting starts suddenly, and whatever is left in the stomach from the last meal is brought up. It can be mild, and the child is quite well otherwise, or more serious with fever and malaise and frequent vomiting over the next twenty-four hours, with nothing but clear fluid and phlegm being brought up.

Herbal teas or tinctures can be given to help resolve the infection quickly and to settle the stomach. (In mild cases, no treatment may be necessary.) Choose from *camomile*, *echinacea*, *lavender*, *lemon balm*, *peppermint* or *thyme*, or give honey water spiced with *ginger* or *cinnamon*. *Garlic* is also very useful.

Frequent vomiting

If the vomiting is very frequent, to help quell the nausea ask the child to suck – not chew – a lozenge or a *slippery elm* tablet for as long as possible, which will help resist the urge to vomit.

Give drinks – herb teas, spring water, dilute apple juice or ginger beer, for example – every few minutes, in sips, to prevent dehydration. Add a pinch of salt and 1 teaspoon (5ml) of glucose per glassful of water, to replace electrolytes lost through vomiting.

Weak Digestion

If the child has a weak stomach, foods will not be digested easily and the stomach will be upset by a number of foods, or combinations of foods. Food allergies may develop. A weak stomach can be constitutional, inherited from a member of the family or related to a difficult birth or to other illness that has lowered the child's vitality because the energy of the body has been concentrated on healing elsewhere. The child may seem lethargic, look pale and thin, and have a pale tongue and a poor appetite. There may be a tendency to constipation or diarrhoea, with particles of undigested food observable in the stools.

It is important to strengthen the stomach using herbs and to respect the child's weakness by giving easily digested foods in small amounts frequently, rather than large meals.

Do not give too much red meat or proteins in the evening, when the digestion is more sluggish anyway.

Avoid excess milk and cut down on sugar.

Warm foods are more easily digested than cold raw foods – vegetable soups and casseroles are better than salads.

Herbs can be given to strengthen the stomach between vomiting attacks. Choose from *cinnamon* and *ginger* made into warm tea and taken three times daily, or *angelica*, *cloves*, *coriander*, *dill*, *fennel*, *hawthorn*, *peppermint*, *sweet flag* and *yarrow*. These can also be used, singly or in combination, and sweetened with honey if you wish.

For vomiting attacks, the same herbs can be used more frequently, given in sips as often as the child wants, and *camomile* can also be used, especially if the child gets upset or distressed.

Emotional Upset

When a child is upset or over-excited, the sympathetic nervous system is on the alert, causing a rush of adrenalin and all the resulting physical changes that accompany stress or excitement, including the flow of energy away from the digestive system. (Digestion works far better when one is relaxed, and the parasympathetic nervous system comes into play.) As a result, the child does not digest properly, the food sits in the stomach, which, if it is very tense, can forcibly throw it out. Children are often prone to vomiting before tests or exams, or if they are anxious or unhappy at school or at home – there is something 'they just can't stomach' or are 'sick and tired of'.

If you feel this is the problem with your child who is prone to vomiting, it is important to talk to the child about any worries and help him or her to learn how to cope with them better and to relax (see Nervous System, page 122). The *Bach Flower Remedies* are extremely useful in these instances and can often work wonders (see page 165).

Relaxing herbs, which soothe the stomach and the nervous system, can be given to the child. These should be given frequently during the vomiting attacks and continued on a more long-term basis between, given three or four times daily until the emotional problem is resolved. Choose from *camomile, catnip, hops, lemon balm, skullcap* or *vervain*.

If the child is very distressed by the vomiting, you can also use Dr Bach's *Rescue Remedy* or another suitable remedy (see Bach Flower Remedies, page 165).

Gastric Catarrh

The lining of the stomach naturally secretes mucus to protect the stomach walls, so that the acid and enzymes digest only the food and do not corrode the sensitive lining. This mucus can become excessive, either through irritation of the stomach from not eating properly or through swallowing mucus from the respiratory system during an infection, such as a cough or a cold. This gives rise to gastric catarrh or phlegm, which stops the stomach from working properly and interferes with the efficient digestion of food. This can give rise to periodic vomiting, as the body tries to clear the phlegm. In this case the vomit is watery and resembles mucus – it can be white, yellow or green. The child will have a stomach ache and feel nauseous, sometimes mildly for a few days, and look pale.

Any catarrhal condition of the respiratory system (see page 93) needs to be resolved.

All mucus-producing foods need to be avoided (see page 94) until the child is better.

Herbal teas can be given to clear the catarrh; choose from *angelica, cardamon, cinnamon, elderflowers, fennel, ginger, meadowsweet* or *peppermint. Golden seal* is one of the best remedies in this instance but, because it is very bitter, you will be able to give it in only small amounts to children. Add 3–5 drops of tincture to your chosen infusion or to a glass of water three times a day.

These remedies can also be used during vomiting attacks, given more frequently in small amounts.

Once the vomiting has stopped and the stomach is working again, give natural live yoghurt with brown rice and garlic to help re-establish the normal bacterial population of the gut.

DIARRHOEA

Causes of Acute Diarrhoea with 'tummy ache'

Acute diarrhoea occurs more commonly in children than vomiting. It tends to last about twenty-four hours and has a number of different causes:

• Over-eating the wrong foods – those that are hard to digest (greasy foods, rich creamy sauces, spices) or even over-indulgence in otherwise healthy foods (such as too much roughage in grains, fruit or vegetables) can irritate the gut and produce loose stools.

• Having too many cold foods and drinks, such as ice-cream, fruit juices and milk from the fridge, salads (especially cucumber, particularly on a hot day), can be a strain on the stomach, which likes to be warm. The child is usually quite well apart from the loose stools.

• Diarrhoea, coupled with vomiting and a mild fever, most commonly could mean gastro-enteritis, food poisoning or, if it is very extreme, dysentery. Often there is an epidemic of diarrhoea going around the community, so that you will easily interpret the symptoms when they come on. Often, mild gastro-enteritis develops when travelling abroad, where it takes the body a while to get used to new foods and different micro-organisms.

- Food poisoning is on the increase, and pre-cooked meals and eggs harbouring organisms, such as listeria and salmonella, are often to blame. There will be fever and often malaise; there could also be nausea and vomiting. If there is vomiting and/or diarrhoea every half hour or so, with mucus or blood in the stools, *call the doctor immediately*.

- If there is another infection – a chest infection, for example – for which the child has been prescribed wide-spectrum antibiotics, this could upset the normal bowel flora and cause resistant organisms to proliferate, causing a mild bowel infection and diarrhoea.

- Stress or over-excitement can cause diarrhoea with tummy aches, both on a short and long-term basis (see Nervous System, page 122).

- If there is diarrhoea with abdominal pain around the umbilicus and to the lower right side, it could indicate appendicitis, *contact your doctor immediately*.

- Diarrhoea often accompanies infections elsewhere in the body, in which case there will be a fever and malaise, as well as other symptoms – a cold, cough or rash, for example.

If there is severe abdominal pain, vomiting and stools containing blood and mucus, it could mean a blocked bowel; contact your doctor immediately.

Causes of Chronic Diarrhoea

This occurs more mildly or periodically than acute diarrhoea.

- It can have several causes, including food allergies, commonly to milk or wheat products (see Allergies, page 67).

- Thread worms (page 140) and candidiasis (page 73) can also cause chronic diarrhoea.

- If a child is run down from other illness, frequent antibiotics or stress, it can weaken the digestion and cause the bowel to be oversensitive to foods and easily irritated and tense, causing diarrhoea.

- If diarrhoea is pale in colour and foul smelling, this could indicate coeliac disease, involving gluten intolerance.

- Involuntary diarrhoea, resulting in a child frequently soiling his or her pants, can be related to chronic constipation. Hard stools can block the bowel, but some liquid stool can get past it once a build-up of faeces occurs.

- Diarrhoea occurs when the intestines are irritated and the bowel muscles contract more frequently and intensely, causing griping and pain, as the body attempts to rid itself of the irritant. The food residues do not stay long enough in the bowel for water and electrolytes to be reabsorbed, so the bowel movement is watery. In the short term, there is a risk of dehydration and temporary electrolyte imbalance; in the long term, there is a risk of additional nutritional disturbance because of chronic poor absorption of vital nutrients.

Treatment of Diarrhoea

Remedies can be given every hour or two in acute diarrhoea and three times daily in chronic cases. If there is a fever, see Fever Management, page 85–8.

Where there is evidence or the possibility of an infection, herbal remedies work very well, as they can treat the bowel whether the infection is viral or bacterial in origin.

Antiseptic Herbs *Garlic* can be given as a natural antibiotic, two perles or 1 teaspoon (5ml) of juice every two or three hours. *Echinacea* can be added to other chosen herbal prescriptions, to help the immune system fight off the infection.

Camomile, thyme, ginger and *fennel* are mildly antiseptic and will help to relax the bowel, relieving griping pains that accompany acute diarrhoea. If the child feels cold and looks pale, *ginger tea* is especially useful as it is very warming. It can also help chronic diarrhoea that is related to low vitality and digestive weakness.

Astringent Herbs For general treatment of diarrhoea, *astringent* herbs can be made into teas or taken in tinctures, and combined with *carminative* herbs to relax the gut and soothe griping and pain.

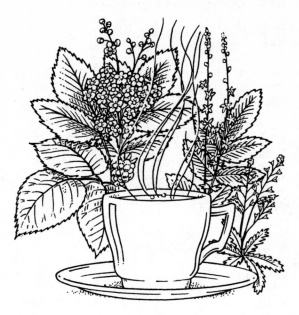

marshmallow, *psyllium seeds* or *slippery elm*. *Slippery elm* can be sucked as tablets, or given as powder made into a gruel by mixing with warm water (and honey if you wish). Add a pinch of *cinnamon* or *ginger* powder.

Essential Oils Dilute 2 drops of *camomile*, *geranium* or *sandalwood* in 1 teaspoon (5ml) of base oil, and massage the abdomen lightly to relax and soothe the digestive tract. *Thyme oil* is very antiseptic and can be added to water and sprayed into the room as a disinfectant, or used in a vaporizer.

Diarrhoea can be a serious condition, particularly for babies and young children. If diarrhoea is frequent it can lead to loss of body fluids and electrolytes and dehydration (see page 88). It is most important to make sure that the child drinks plenty – if they only want liquid in sips, give it frequently.

Recipe to Counteract Dehydration

This is a useful recipe to help replace lost electrolytes:

$\frac{1}{2}$ teaspoon (2–3ml) common salt (sodium chloride)
$\frac{1}{4}$ teaspoon (1–2ml) sodium bicarbonate (soda)
$\frac{1}{4}$ teaspoon (1–2ml) potassium chloride
2 tablespoons (40ml) glucose

Add the above to 2 pints (1 litre) of water and mix it to equal parts of herbal tea, made from *peppermint* and *fennel* or *ginger*, and give as frequently as possible.

Dietary Treatment for Diarrhoea

If there is acute diarrhoea, particularly with fever, it is best to give no food or milk – just fluids – and to fast the child for a few hours.

- Once the appetite has returned and the child feels a little better, you can give blackberries, strawberries, apples or pears or juices of these, as they have astringent properties which help contain the diarrhoea. These are best given warm, as cold foods should be avoided as much as possible.

- Astringent herbs include *agrimony*, *blackberry leaves*, *geranium* (*cranesbill*), *meadowsweet*, *oakbark*, *shepherd's purse* and *tormentil*. *Carminative herbs* include *cardamon*, *cinnamon*, *fennel*, *ginger* and *peppermint*.

- A useful prescription, which I give frequently, is to mix equal parts of *agrimony* and *tormentil* with a pinch of *ginger* or *cinnamon*. Unsweetened blackcurrant juice is delicious and contains astringent tannins and a high vitamin C content. A glass can be taken several times daily.

- Lemon juice will help to astringe the gut and can be very pleasant and effective when combined with *ginger*. Simmer $\frac{1}{4}$ teaspoon (1–2ml) chopped or grated ginger in a cup of water for 5 minutes. Add the juice of half a lemon and 1 teaspoon (5ml) of honey.

- *Arrowroot* powder can also be taken.

Demulcent Herbs Soothing demulcent herbs will help to calm the irritated gut lining and are easily digested and nutritious. One or two should be added to prescriptions of astringent, carminative and antiseptic herbs. Choose from *comfrey*, *Iceland moss*, *linseed*,

- Brown rice, cooked until it is very soft, can be given mixed with honey, and natural live yoghurt can be given with mashed banana to help re-establish the normal bacterial population of the gut and to prevent further infection.

- Sprigs of *mint* can be added to rice or yoghurt to calm the stomach and quell any griping.

- You can make an interesting beverage from: $\frac{1}{2}$ cup live yoghurt, $\frac{1}{2}$ cup water, 1 teaspoon (5ml) of fresh grated *nutmeg* and a pinch of *ginger* and *cinnamon*.

Once the bowel has completely settled down, normal eating can be resumed. Keep meals regular and do not let the child eat between meals or eat cold foods to help recovery of the digestive tract. Give easily digestible meals and no junk food.

FOOD POISONING

If you suspect food poisoning, you can give the child an emetic, using a strong solution of *mustard* – 1 teaspoon (5ml) of dry mustard in 3 tablespoons (60ml) of tepid water.

- You can use other things, which act as neutralizing agents and also to help rid the body of the toxins:

☐ Cider vinegar – 1 teaspoon (5ml) in a glass of water, give sips every 5 minutes
☐ 1 cup of miso soup with $\frac{1}{2}$ teaspoon (2–3ml) each of *coriander* and *cumin* seeds
☐ Strong *liquorice* tea
☐ Milk and honey

DYSENTERY

This is a more severe type of diarrhoea, caused by irritation and inflammation of the bowel lining from infection by *Shigella bacillus*. Symptoms include griping abdominal pains, fever, nausea and/or vomiting, lethargy and malaise, and diarrhoea with mucus, pus or blood, passed very frequently, possibly every 30 minutes or so.

Dysentery is rare in this climate, but it can occur from travelling abroad or from areas of poor sanitation. Children are particularly prone if their already toxic bowels present an ideal breeding ground for the germs.

If you suspect dysentery, especially in a small child, call your doctor.

Treatment of Dysentry

Most importantly, administer plenty of fluids as frequently as possible.

- Useful herbs include *American cranesbill, bayberry, gum arabic, nettles, shepherd's purse* and *tormentil*, while *camomile, dill, fennel, ginger* and *peppermint* soothe griping.

- *Garlic* capsules should be given frequently to help re-establish normal gut flora. *Echinacea* will help enhance the immune response to the infection.

- Mix equal parts of *bayberry* and *raspberry* leaves with $\frac{1}{2}$ part of *ginger* or *cinnamon*. Use 2–3 teaspoons (10–15ml) per cup of boiling water, and give every few hours until there is an improvement.

- Give raw carrot juice, lemon and honey, apple juice or lemon and water.

- While symptoms are acute, give no solid food.

- Once the appetite returns (after 24 hours or so) give live natural yoghurt and brown rice. Also apples, blackberries, pears and strawberries, which are all astringent and help allay irritation of the gut and diarrhoea.

- *Slippery elm* gruel with honey is also useful.

If symptoms are severe, or do not clear within 24 hours, seek professional help. Call your doctor immediately if: the child seems listless or the limbs are floppy, the eyes look sunken, the urine is dark and concentrated or there is weight loss, as this will indicate dehydration.

HICCUPS

Frequent bouts of hiccups suggest either a fatty diet or a weak or disturbed digestion.

Food could be fermenting in the stomach through poor digestion or wrong combinations of foods – acid fruit with carbohydrate, for example – causing a build-up of gas or phlegm. Drinking too much liquid with foods can dilute the digestive juices and cause poor breakdown of food, leading to fermentation and irritation of the stomach. The irritation and fermentation in the stomach causes spasm of the diaphragm, which cause the characteristic jerks or hiccups.

Treatment of Hiccups

Treatment is aimed at relaxing the stomach and diaphragm with carminative herbs, while stimulating digestion at the same time.

• Herbs such as *aniseed, catnip, dill, fennel, ginger* and *lavender* are all indicated.

• Freshly grated or desiccated coconut mixed with equal parts of honey is also helpful.

TRAVEL SICKNESS

Nausea and/or vomiting can be due to motion sickness brought about by the motion of a car, boat or plane, disturbing the balance mechanism in the inner ear. The eyes are also important to our sense of balance, so that, when the inner ears sense the motion of the vehicle but the eyes are looking at something different – such as reading or playing in the car – there is some confusion about the two different messages from the balance mechanism to the brain, which sets off nausea or vomiting. It can be exacerbated by nervousness or apprehension about the journey, as well as exhaust fumes from traffic.

Treatment of Travel Sickness

• Encourage the child to keep looking out of the window, at the horizon or the passing countryside to prevent too much time spent looking down. This is easily done by inventing games that involve the child looking for things through the window – letter boxes, different types of cars, animals and so on.

• Make sure there is plenty of fresh air – keep the car window open a little and take walks on deck on a boat.

• The neiguan point on the wrist can be massaged (see Figure 13) or sea bands, which exert pressure on the point, can be worn. This prevents nausea.

• *Ginger* is a wonderful remedy for travel sickness. It can be taken as crystallized ginger, and chewed as a preventative before a journey, or when nausea arises. Ginger can be ground into food taken before or during a journey. Home-made ginger biscuits, ginger beer, dilute ginger tincture or ginger tea can all be used.

• Other herbs may also prove effective. *Camomile, fennel, lemon balm, meadowsweet* and *peppermint* will all help to settle the stomach, and can be taken frequently in the form of teas.

• Essential oils of *aniseed, cinnamon, fennel, ginger, melissa* or *peppermint* can be inhaled. Put a few drops on a handkerchief or cotton wool or on clothes.

CHRONIC INTERMITTENT STOMACH ACHES

There are a number of causes of nagging stomach aches in children, which come and go: constipation, worms, food intolerance (see Allergies, page 67), including coeliac disease, stress or psychological problems (see Nervous System, page 122), infection elsewhere in the body, or appendicitis.

CONSTIPATION

Most children have at least one bowel movement every day, sometimes two. If they do not, they are suffering from constipation, and this can cause stomach aches which often occur around meal times.

Causes of Constipation

Constipation in children can be simply the

result of poor bowel habits. If the urge to pass a stool is ignored by a child who is in a hurry to eat breakfast and rush off to school, or by a toddler too engrossed in play, it may be another 24 hours before another chance occurs. Very often, even if the call to stool is heeded, the child may still be too preoccupied to take enough time to evacuate properly, and a residue remains, which gradually builds up more and more and, as it stays in the large bowel, so it loses moisture and becomes harder to pass. Once a child has experienced the painful passing of a hard stool, he or she will feel even more reluctant to do so again.

• Constipation can also be due to poor diet, excess animal protein causing putrefaction in the bowel, too much over-refined foods – white bread, white flour, cakes and biscuits, for example and not enough roughage in whole grains, fruit and vegetables.

• Exercise is required to promote healthy circulation of blood to the bowel muscles for them to work efficiently. Too little exercise, perhaps too much sitting around watching television, can contribute to constipation.

• Specific food intolerance – to wheat, gluten or milk produce – can irritate the gut, causing tension and spasm of bowel muscles, inhibiting peristaltic bowel movements.

• If a child is ill or feverish or if there has been vomiting, causing loss of water from the body, the bowel compensates by absorbing water from the stools. This is not true constipation, only a temporary state, as the bowels return to normal once the child feels better.

• Worry, anxiety, in fact, stresses of all kinds, can produce tension in the bowel muscles, causing 'spastic' constipation. This might occur during transition from one phase of life to another – starting play school, moving to secondary school, for instance – and the child may feel insecure and is 'holding on', in this case to the stool.

• Vitamin and mineral deficiencies can play a part in erratic bowel movements, particularly vitamin C and magnesium deficiency and aluminium excess.

• If a child does not regularly drink enough fluid, this can cause a hard, dry stool which is difficult to pass.

The auto-intoxication that results from constipation can cause lethargy, poor concentration, irritability, poor sleeping habits, headaches and muscle aches.

Treatment of Constipation

Treatment will obviously depend to some extent on the cause of the constipation. If this is difficult to determine, you may need to call on professional help. However, there are some general measures.

• Every call to stool needs to be heeded, but this may be difficult to explain to your small child. The best thing to do is to put the child on the potty or loo at regular times through the day after meals, so that at least they get the opportunity should the urge occur. Older children will understand more easily and can be taught to take the time needed for a proper bowel movement every day – perhaps by getting up ten minutes earlier to avoid the rush in the morning!

• The diet should contain plenty of fruit and vegetables, raw or lightly cooked with their skins, and whole grains, nuts and seeds to provide sufficient fibre to bulk out the stool and encourage evacuation as well as discourage the growth of putrefactive bacteria. Figs, prunes, raisins, apricots, desiccated coconut, rhubarb, watercress, parsley and honey are all especially helpful.

• You can help balance intestinal bacteria by giving the child plenty of live yoghurt, olive oil and *garlic* (raw or in juice or perles). Anything other than ripe banana (which actively encourages beneficial bacteria) added to the yoghurt will actually destroy many of the benign bacteria. Alternatively, acidophilus tablets can be given to help to improve transit time of food through the bowel by balancing the intestinal bacteria in the same way.

• When adding roughage to the diet, do not give the child, especially if he or she is aged three or under, too much bran or brown bread, which are difficult to digest and can actually act as a bowel irritant, slowing down bowel activity and so aggravating constipation. Wheat bran can be particularly difficult, especially since many children have a specific food intolerance to wheat. Wheat is probably the most allergenic food there is, and it can be implicated in constipation and abdominal pain among a variety of other symptoms (see Allergies, page 67).

• Gluten allergies may also occur in children, not necessarily as frank coeliac disease (see page 141), but causing a variety of bowel problems. Gluten is found in wheat, oats, barley and rye. Milk allergies can also be involved.

• Encourage your child to play outside or take regular and active exercise, such as swimming, bicycling, riding, walking and dancing.

Herbal Laxatives

It is not a good idea to give laxatives as the sole means of treatment to a child, because their bowels, like those of an adult, may become habituated to their use. However, to soften the stools and evacuate hard, impacted faeces and to cleanse the system, they can be used in the short term, as long as attention is paid to background causes, such as diet and bowel habits, as well as any emotional problems, to remedy the situation for good.

Bulk Laxative Herbs Herbs that help moisten and bulk out the bowel contents and push them along include *psyllium seeds* and *flax seeds*. Take 1 teaspoon (5ml) in a cup of warm water. Allow to swell into a gel and take before bed.

Stimulating Herbs Other herbs are stimulating to the bowels and are particularly useful for children who tend to be weak, sluggish or sedentary and their bowel muscles rather inactive. They are also useful for sluggish liver function because they help to stimulate bile secretion, which helps produce a normal bowel movement. These include *butternut, cascara, dandelion root, liquorice root* and *yellow dock root*. These can be made into decoctions and sweetened with honey, or 5–10 drops of tincture can be taken in water three times daily.

Soothing Herbs These herbs contain muci-

lage, which attracts water and so helps to moisten the stool and acts as a lubricant, helping to clear the gut of hard impacted stools. They include *slippery elm*, which can be taken as tablets or a powder made into a gruel by mixing with equal parts of water and a pinch of *cinnamon* or *ginger* powder, and *comfrey root*, which can be made into a decoction and added to other herbs; this is very useful to heal and repair tissues where the gut has been irritated and weakened.

Relaxing Herbs Some herbs can be given for a tense, over-contracted bowel, which may occur in a tense, anxious or over-active child. These include *camomile, fennel, ginger, peppermint, valerian* and *wild yam*. Once the bowel muscles are relaxed, normal peristaltic bowel movements should occur more easily.

When you make a prescription for your child's constipation, choose a predominance of herbs from the category you think is most suitable but combine them with at least one from the other groups. A useful recipe is to prepare *camomile, comfrey root, dandelion root, liquorice sticks, peppermint* and *wild yam* as a decoction and give three times daily. Sweeten with honey.

• A teaspoon of honey or molasses in a cup of hot water first thing in the morning is a tasty and very nutritious remedy for mild constipation. Children love it. Honey and lemon can also be given on rising if preferred. Alternatively, apricots mashed with a little honey are delicious and highly effective.

• Massage to the abdomen is a lovely way to treat your child's constipation, and touch is particularly beneficial when the child is feeling anxious or insecure. You can use dilute essential oils of *camomile, fennel, lavender* or *rosemary*. Always massage in the direction of the bowel movements – clockwise.

• If you find that laxative herbs need to be given to your child on a regular basis, you are not reaching the root cause of the problem. There may be food intolerance, in which case you can eliminate one suspected food at a time – wheat or milk, for example – for three or four weeks to ascertain a clear picture. There may be other less obvious problems, and it is best to seek advice from a professional herbalist.

If a child has not passed a stool for four days, if the abdomen becomes distended or painful or if the child becomes lethargic or particularly distressed, take him or her to the doctor immediately – there may be a blockage of the bowel.

WORMS

These can occur frequently in children. There are three types of worms: threadworms, round worms and tapeworms (which require professional help).

Threadworms

These are about ½in (1cm) long and are the most common type in children of temperate climates, particularly in children aged between two and six, when they can spend much time with dirty fingers in their mouths!

Worms live in the large intestine and rectum and give rise to anal itching, particularly at night. They can also cause disturbed sleep, tooth grinding, bad dreams, constipation and/ or diarrhoea, abdominal pain, bad breath, poor or increased appetite, lethargy and dark rings under the eyes, dry skin on the cheeks and nose picking.

The life-cycle of the threadworm helps to explain how infection is caught and passed on. When the female worm is ready to lay eggs, it migrates from the large intestine to the rectum and anus, and lays its eggs at night – this activity causes the itching. It then goes back to the intestine. The itching causes the child to scratch, and the eggs are carried on the fingers, under finger nails. If the child then sucks its fingers or thumb, or bites its nails, the eggs are ingested, and they pass into the intestine where they hatch. They can also cause inflammation in the part of the bowel to which they attach. A worm lives for six to eight weeks. If the child touches clothes, toys etc. they become contaminated with eggs, which are easily passed on among family and playmates.

If you suspect that your child has worms, look carefully at the anus an hour or so after bed, or apply a proprietary clear adhesive tape to the anus and peel it off in the morning to examine for eggs. The threadworm will look like a tiny piece of white thread. Worms can sometimes be seen in the stools. If your child has worms, it is sensible to treat any other children in the family and any pets, as they can pass them on. If you are unsure, you can take a stool sample to the doctor for laboratory analysis.

Round Worms

These are rarer, being found mostly in tropical climates or in an environment where hygiene is poor. Greatest risk occurs when travelling abroad.

The worms are pale yellow or white and can measure 4–5in (10–13cm) in length. Several can live in the intestine at once, putting more strain on a child's health than the smaller threadworms. They lay eggs in the duodenum (small intestine) and can multiply quickly, causing abdominal pain, which is often severe, diarrhoea, vomiting, poor appetite and coughing, as the worms can migrate to the lungs, and the child will not thrive and will lose weight.

Not all children get worms, and this is related to effective function of the digestive tract. If the digestive enzymes are secreted in full strength and with regular peristaltic movements, which means good bowel habits to keep the bowel healthy, there is less likelihood of them thriving.

Treatment of Worms

• Foods and herbs can be given that are toxic to worms. These include: *garlic* (give one or two cloves chopped finely in a spoonful of honey or in a little warm milk 30 minutes before breakfast), raw onions, pumpkin seeds, raw carrots and carrot juice, cayenne pepper (added to cooking or in yoghurt), apples, desiccated coconut and raw turnip.

• Try giving ground pumpkin seeds in grated carrot for breakfast.

• Useful herbs include *wormwood, southernwood, balmony, gentian, vervain* and, *pennyroyal* (none of these should be taken by pregnant women), and *sage, peppermint, thyme, aniseed, blue flag, fennel, self-heal* and *echinacea*. When treating older children, add a tiny pinch of

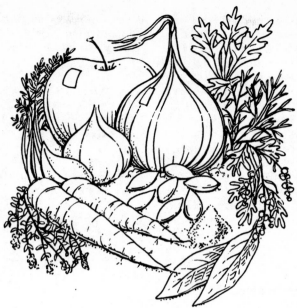

cayenne (or, if using *cayenne* tincture, 1 or 2 drops) to teas.

● Many of the anthelmintic (to expel worms) herbs are strong and bitter tasting. They can be added to more aromatic herbs, such as *fennel* and *peppermint*, and sweetened with a little honey. They are best taken first thing in the morning, a cupful or so at a time, on an empty stomach so that they have more impact in the intestine before they are diluted by food, and then two or three times again through the day before meals. Repeat for a week. If you cannot persuade your child to take a whole cupful, give sips as frequently as possible through the day, or dilute in juice.

● A useful recipe is to make tea from
1 part *chelone*
1 part *peppermint*
½ part *wormwood*
1 part *aniseed*.
Alternatively, the herbs can be powdered in a coffee grinder and given in a teaspoonful of honey or molasses. Check stools for expelled worms.

● Other laxative foods, and herbs such as *liquorice* or *dandelion root*, can be given to speed the expulsion of the worms from the intestines.

● Repeat treatment after two weeks to ensure expulsion of those worms that were eggs or just hatched at the time of the initial treatment.

● Pay particular attention to your children's hygiene. Explain to them the importance of washing their hands frequently, in hot, soapy water especially before eating and after touching pets, and try to persuade them not to scratch an itchy bottom. Closely fitted underwear or pyjamas at night will help to prevent them. Scrub fingernails every day.

● Avoid giving sweets and sugary foods and refined carbohydrates, as worms thrive on these. Give live yoghurt daily to enhance bowel health and to discourage putrefaction.

● *Calendula ointment* or a couple of drops of essential oils – *eucalyptus*, *lavender*, *tea tree*, *thyme*, for example – in petroleum jelly can be applied to the anus at night to prevent the worms from laying eggs and to relieve the itching.

FOOD INTOLERANCE AND ALLERGY
(See also page 67)

Coeliac Disease

This is a condition in which the intestine has a sensitivity to (or intolerance of) gluten, a protein found in wheat, oats, barley and rye. It is not a common problem and tends to occur less

141

in breast-fed babies and in children who have not been given gluten-containing cereals at too young an age. It is best to wait until the baby is ten or twelve months old before giving them these.

The inflammation produced in the gut leads to malabsorption, as the irritated villi in the small intestine atrophy and reduce the surface area for food absorption. This is a serious problem as it severely compromises nutrition and results in failure to thrive and loss of weight, lethargy, anaemia, mineral and vitamin deficiencies and vague symptoms of ill-health.

Other symptoms include diarrhoea, distension of the abdomen, wind and colic; there may be some vomiting, poor appetite, irritability and pale, bulky, smelly stools.

Treatment of Coeliac Disease

Since all gluten has to be avoided, other grains need to be substituted – brown rice, millet and buckwheat, for example – and potatoes, pulses and beans can be eaten freely. (Gluten-free cookery books are obtainable from health food shops and book stores.) Removing gluten from the diet allows the gut to function normally again, and the child will begin to recover and thrive again.

• Herbal remedies can be given to soothe the irritated intestinal lining and to help repair the damage. These include *agrimony*, *camomile*, *comfrey*, *marshmallow*, *slippery elm* and *wild yam*.

• Nutritional deficiencies will need to be made up through an excellent diet and mineral and vitamin supplements.

Malabsorption

This is caused not only by coeliac disease and gluten sensitivity, but also by a range of other food intolerances, which can reduce the small intestine's ability to absorb nourishment. Other food allergens frequently affecting children are milk products (milk, cheese, butter, cream, yoghurt, ice-cream and foods containing them), sugar and eggs. If you suspect any of these foods, eliminate them for three or four weeks. If you are on the right track, symptoms such as bloating and wind, diarrhoea/constipation and abdominal discomfort, irritability and lethargy should have diminished.

Treatment of Malabsorption

Herbal remedies can be taken to soothe and repair the gut lining.

• *Comfrey*, *Iceland moss*, *marshmallow* and *slippery elm* are soothing and healing to the mucous membranes.

• *Camomile*, *meadowsweet* and *wild yam* are anti-inflammatory and healing.

• *Agrimony* and *tormentil* are astringent to aid healing.

INFECTION CAUSING ABDOMINAL PAIN

Very often infection elsewhere, particularly in the respiratory tract – catarrh, coughs and tonsilitis, for instance – can cause abdominal pain, which can be either acute and painful, or recurrent and milder. The lymph nodes in and around the intestine sometimes become tender and swollen as lymphocytes multiply to fight off infection, viruses or bacteria, which have been swallowed or which are in the bloodstream. This is known as mesenteric adenitis. The most important thing in this case is to clear up the original infection and the swollen lymph nodes will disappear (see Respiratory Tract, page 89).

Cystitis can also cause lower abdominal pain and can either be acute or a low-grade urinary infection. In most cases there will be other signs of bladder inflammation, such as frequency of urination, pain passing water, poor appetite, pale face, crying and generally feeling unwell (see Urinary System, page 154).

APPENDICITIS

Another cause of acute and recurrent abdominal pain is appendicitis. The appendix is situated on the right side of the abdomen, and it is a small, worm-shaped attachment to the caecum (the beginning of the large intestine) about $2\frac{3}{4}$in (7cm) long. It can become inflamed

Symptoms of Acute Appendicitis

- ☐ Severe pain in the centre and radiating to the lower right of the abdomen
- ☐ nausea and/or vomiting
- ☐ diarrhoea
- ☐ raised temperature
- ☐ rapid pulse
- ☐ a coated tongue
- ☐ bad breath

and infected when blocked by impacted faeces.

When the inflammation arises, it produces recurring abdominal pains, which are colicky in nature, around the umbilicus, as well as loss of appetite, nausea and sometimes vomiting. As the condition worsens, the pain and colic radiate further out and become more intense. An inflamed appendix can 'grumble' away for some time, months or even years, in this way, during which time it can be treated with diet and herbal remedies. However, if you suspect a 'grumbling appendix', always seek professional help.

This is a very serious condition, which can lead to peritonitis (when the appendix bursts), and it requires urgent medical attention.

Treatment of Appendicitis

If you suspect a 'grumbling appendix', there may be other conditions in the bowel that are affecting it and causing the blockage and inflammation of the appendix. Diagnosis and treatment will need professional help. It may be that there is constipation, wind, irritation from food intolerance, anxiety or stress causing tension in the bowel, or inflammation of lymph nodes around the intestine related to a respiratory infection, such as tonsilitis (mesenteric adenitis).

- To help resolve the inflammation and irritation and the toxic state of the bowels, the following herbs are useful: *agrimony, camomile, echinacea, liquorice* and *wild yam*. These can be combined together in a decoction and taken three times daily, over several months if necessary.

- Appendicitis is seen less commonly in people who have plenty of roughage in their diet from fruit and vegetables, whole grains, nuts and seeds. In general, follow the advice given for constipation (page 138), but never use laxatives, which may aggravate the problem.

THE SKIN

The outer covering to our bodies is intricately designed to fulfil a variety of different functions. It is our first line of defence against damage from infection, chemical pollution, extremes of temperature and light, and physical injury. It secretes antiseptic substances to ward off invading micro-organisms, and is also inhabited by beneficial bacteria as a back-up in defence, discouraging proliferation of more unfavourable ones. For this reason, it is important that the skin is not disturbed overmuch by antiseptic creams, perfumes, deodorants and so on. When it is very cold, blood vessels in the skin contract and keep the heat inside the body to prevent it becoming too cold; when it is very hot, these blood vessels dilate, and the blood suffuses to the surface of the body, allowing it to lose heat into the atmosphere, and thereby keep the body cool.

The skin is also a major organ of excretion via its several million sweat glands. The average adult excretes about 1 pint (600ml) of fluid a day through the skin; during vigorous exercise or in very hot weather this can increase ten times or more. Sweat contains water, mineral salts, nitrogenous wastes and other toxins, and it is similar in content to urine. This pathway of excretion is put to great use by herbalists who use diaphoretic herbs – *camomile, catnip, limeflowers* and *yarrow*, for example – to increase perspiration and thereby clear toxins from the system, as well as bring down a fever. Sweat forms a protective acid covering to the body, helping to ward off harmful bacteria. When a child does not take sufficient vigorous exercise to produce a sweat on a regular basis, this puts a great burden on the other organs of elimination (the lungs, bowels and kidneys),

143

which may account for chronic problems such as catarrh and sinusitis and tonsilitis.

The skin plays a major part in maintaining a stable inner environment in another way – it regulates the water and electrolyte balance in the body by its composition of sweat and in this way works hand in hand with the kidneys. Thus, not only will it excrete unwanted substances and toxins, but it will also protect against the loss of vital body fluids.

The skin is an organ of sense: it is richly supplied with sensitive nerve endings, which relay messages to the brain about sensations from the outside world – heat or cold, pleasure or pain. It is our point of contact between our inner and our outer worlds, so we may hardly be surprised that many skin diseases arise not only through physical abuse of the skin, from polluted air or chemicals in creams, but also through emotional disharmony. The skin reflects our inner state on both physical and emotional levels, and this is apparent to us all – we can observe the pale pinched face of a frightened child and the rosy lustre on the cheeks of a happy bouncy child, a healthy glow of the skin in a healthy child, or the sallow complexion of a sick child. It is a useful diagnostic aid, which you can easily use with your children.

A wide variety of skin problems develop in children. Some are very much related to a child's emotional state – rashes and eczema, for example: others are due to external factors – chemicals, wounds or sunburn, for instance; while the rest are either due to the body's inability to cope with external factors, such as sensitivity to plants, allergy to foods, or infections such as impetigo and scabies. The skin's ability to deal with these factors depends very much on the nutrients brought to the skin by the underlying blood vessels. Deficiencies of certain minerals, vitamins and trace elements can impair the skin's resilience and lead to a number of skin disorders. A healthy skin, for example, will not allow impetigo to proliferate because its local immune mechanisms will be fully operational. An impaired skin function will allow such an infection to spread, because it will be unable to rally its defences sufficiently to beat it without outside help. Healthy skin function is also dependent on an efficient circulation of blood, which brings nutrients to the skin and carries away the waste products of metabolism.

ECZEMA

Eczema is an itchy skin condition in which the skin becomes red and inflamed. There are many variations in the state of the skin. Sometimes there are small bubbles just beneath the skin, which can burst to produce a weeping rash; this can then form dry-looking crusts. Other times there may be a dry, scaly, red rash. If the eczema is long standing, it can present as dry, scaly, hard and thickened skin. If it is particularly dry, the skin can easily crack and bleed. Naturally any child will want to scratch an itchy skin, and this may introduce infection, particularly herpes and staphylococcus, into broken skin, causing further inflammation. Where eczema occurs in the nappy area, it is particularly prone to secondary thrush (monilia) infection.

Eczema is an allergic condition. It can be atopic eczema, which usually develops when a baby is a few months old, particularly around the same time as the introduction of solid foods, and it begins as an itchy, dry, red rash on the face, neck, nappy area, hands and creases of the arms and legs. It is common for this type of eczema to be followed by other allergic reactions, such as asthma and hay fever.

Seborrhoeic eczema occurs in the areas of the skin where sebaceous glands are concentrated, such as the scalp (particularly in small babies, see Cradle Cap, page 47), the eyelashes and eyelids, the external ear canal, around the ear, the nose and in the groin.

Ezcema can be triggered by a number of different foods – particularly dairy produce, eggs and wheat – also by external irritants such as biological washing powders, perfumes, wool and animal fur. Emotional upset or stress of any kind can also cause or aggravate the condition. It may be that the eruption of the skin is a means of expression of some internal, perhaps otherwise hidden feelings.

Eczema tends to occur more in bottle-fed babies or children than those who were breast-fed. Breast milk contains many components necessary for the normal development and function of a child's immune system, such as gamma linoleic acid, which formula milks do not. It is particularly important for children with a family history of eczema, asthma or hay fever, to be breast-fed exclusively for three or four months, for even one exposure to cow's milk can set off an allergic response.

Conditions Which Aggravate Eczema

Some substances or conditions can aggravate eczema; these vary from one child to another:

☐ Sweating is aggravated by the use of synthetic fibres next to the skin and by heat, so do not overdress the child, particularly at night, and avoid synthetic bedclothes.

☐ Wool – always use cotton next to the skin.

☐ Soaps and detergents – never wash the skin with soap and avoid using biological detergents. It may be best to wash all underclothes in *pure* soap (flakes or liquid).

☐ Water, especially if it is very chlorinated, can irritate and dry out the skin. Oil, such as olive oil or almond oil, can be added to the bath water, and creams can be used after a bath to keep a dry skin moist.

☐ Scratching an itchy skin will only make it worse or introduce infection. Try putting gloves on a baby or toddler at night, cover all itchy areas with dressings or clothes that cannot easily be removed, and make sure that fingernails are kept cut short and clean.

☐ Vaccinations place further stress on the immune system and can seriously aggravate eczema. Discuss this with your doctor, especially before giving smallpox and tetanus injections.

☐ Cold – eczema is often worse in the winter, perhaps because of the dryness of heated houses, lack of circulation and air to the skin and heavy winter clothes.

☐ Eczema can be related not only to an inherited susceptibility but also to nutritional deficiencies of certain food substances that are vital for the immune system. Most frequently it is related to a disturbance of the metabolism of essential fatty acids, caused by deficiency of unrefined oils and excess of refined oils and saturated fats, sugar and additives in the diet. Deficiencies of zinc, B vitamins, calcium and magnesium are also often responsible.

General Treatment of Eczema

• It is important to establish as far as possible the cause of your child's eczema so that you can treat it effectively.

• If the immune system is not coping well with certain substances – eggs, milk and so on – it is important to identify them and remove them for a limited period while you treat the child and then gradually reintroduce them (see Food Allergies, page 141). Other culprit foods may include wheat, tomatoes, citrus fruits, blackcurrants, sugar, chocolate, yeast extract, pork, beef, peppers and aubergines.

• If there is a familial tendency to allergy, it may be that the inherited weakness in the immune system needs to be treated on a long-term basis, particularly by providing nutritional support in the form of supplements, including B complex, vitamin C, a multi-mineral and vitamin and *evening primrose oil*. Make sure that there are plenty of unrefined oils in the diet every day, including oils from nuts and seeds, beans and pulses, fatty fish (for instance by giving cod liver oil) and virgin vegetable oils (olive, sunflower, safflower and so on). Avoid the use of refined oils, excess saturated fats and sugar and avoid all food additives. Give the child plenty of fresh fruit and vegetables every day.

• If the allergic tendency has been brought to light by stress or emotional upset, this may need to be sorted out within the family, and you may need to give extra love, support and reassurance to a child who is struggling to accept changes from one phase of life to another. You way want to use *Bach Flower Remedies* (see page 165) or herbs for the nervous system (see page 125) to help you through difficult times.

• Sleeping can be a problem if the skin is particularly itchy, and eczema often gets worse at night. If a child becomes tired and run down through lack of sleep, it will only make the problem worse (see Herbs for Insomnia, page 128).

• If a child is particularly anxious it is important not to disclose your anxiety about them or their skin to them, for this will only exacerbate the problem. A child with bad eczema at school may be teased or singled out, and this may require very sensitive handling, including, perhaps, a talk with the school teacher.

Herbal Treatment of Eczema

• The herbal treatment for eczema is aimed mainly at correcting the internal imbalance that is giving rise to the external symptoms. Herbs to support the immune system, such as *camomile*, *echinacea*, *nettles*, *red clover* and *yarrow* can be combined with herbs to support the adrenal glands, such as *borage*, *liquorice* and *wild yam*. These are particularly useful if steroid creams have been used and you want to reduce them gradually.

• Herbs to cool and nourish the blood need to be included in any prescription. Choose from *burdock*, *fumitory*, *heartsease*, *nettles* and *red clover*.

• If there is anxiety or stress, add herbs to support the nervous system, such as *camomile*, *skullcap*, *vervain* and *wild oats*.

• Herbs to treat eczema are always better taken as teas rather than as tinctures. A useful prescription to be given as tea at least three times daily is made from equal parts of *borage*, *burdock root*, *camomile*, *nettles* and *peppermint*.

• At the same time, herbs can be used externally to help resolve inflammation or infection and to restore normal skin function. To moisturize dry skin use almond oil or olive oil with a few drops of essential oil of *camomile* or *lemon balm* (melissa) – add 2 drops to 1 teaspoon (5ml) of oil. This can also be used as a bath oil. Alternatively you can use *evening primrose oil*, vitamin E oil or *aloe vera gel*.

• If the skin is weeping or infected, instead of oils, you can try adding sea salt or cider vinegar to the bath, or a strong infusion of *marigold flowers* in the bath or as a compress, which should be applied frequently through the day, depending on the severity of the problem.

• To reduce the inflammation use compresses of *burdock root*, *chickweed*, *coltsfoot leaf*, *comfrey*, *golden seal*, *marigold*, *witch hazel* or *yellow dock*.

• Alternatively, you could use creams or ointments. Creams can be used particularly if the skin is oozing and weepy, while ointments can be used where the skin is dry.

• A simple cream can be made using aqueous cream (available from chemists), into which you can stir small amounts of a strong infusion of any of the above herbs, or a few drops of essential oil of *camomile* or *lemon balm* (melissa). Use 3–5 drops to 2fl oz (50ml of cream). Moistened oatmeal applied to the skin can also be effective. Ointments can be easily made (see page 27) from the same herbs, and ointments or creams can be applied frequently through the day.

• To aid the cleansing process, make sure that you give the child plenty of fresh fruit and vegetables and laxative foods (see page 138).

Use of Steroid Creams

The use of steroid creams is widespread and, although they may substantially reduce the inflammation, they do not resolve the underlying problem, but merely suppress the external expression of inner imbalance and push it into the body, often to the lungs, where it can lead to asthma later on. Steroid creams are absorbed through the skin, and they may have a suppressive effect on the body's ability to produce natural cortisone. They can also cause a thinning of the skin, making it more susceptible to irritation and to a breakdown of its normal function.

• If your child has been using hydrocortisone cream frequently, it will be necessary to reduce it gradually, or an acute flare-up may result and cause distress.

• Use the herbal cream and steroid creams alternately to begin with, and gradually increase the herbal and reduce the steroid cream. How slowly you need to do this will depend entirely on the individual child.

• Eczema can be interpreted as a cleansing effort on the part of the body, a throwing out of poisons that are not being properly eliminated elsewhere. Hydrocortisone cream simply pushes these poisons into the body.

If your child's eczema does not improve within two or three months of applying the above measures, consult a herbal practitioner for further guidance.

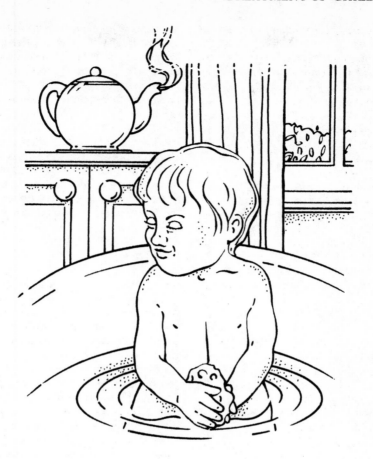

HIVES (URTICARIA OR NETTLE RASH)

This is an allergic skin reaction, caused mostly by eating certain foods or by taking medicine to which the child is sensitive, such as citrus fruit, milk produce, strawberries, chocolate, tomatoes, fish (especially shell fish), foods high in salicylates, nuts, artificial colourings, aspirin and penicillin. It can sometimes result from contact with substances such as animal dander, pollen, make-up, creams, insect stings, and even strong sunlight.

The reaction causes a rash similar to a nettle sting. The eruptions have a red base and white lumps on top, which can be itchy. The rash can affect any area of the body, but if it affects the mouth or lips it can lead to swelling of the tongue or throat (known as angio-neurotic oedema), which can cause serious breathing or swallowing problems. Should this develop, call the doctor immediately. Sometimes the skin rash can be accompanied by joint pains.

Very often hives occur and disappear again within a few hours of exposure to the allergen, and it is quite clear which substance the child is allergic to – too many strawberries, for example. However, some children have frequent attacks or bouts of hives, which can last for weeks. It is important to identify the allergen and remove it, but if the attack is long lasting there may be more than one substance involved or there may be a reaction to a fungal infection (candida), and it will require more thorough treatment of the immune system to resolve the allergic tendency.

Treatment of Hives

A warm herbal bath will help to relieve the itching and inflammation in an acute reaction. Make a strong infusion of *wild pansy* and *fumitory* or *burdock* and *chickweed* and pour it into a hot bath. Soak the child for at least half an hour.

147

• Alternatively, you can make a strong decoction of equal parts of *burdock root*, *fumitory*, *golden seal* and *yellow dock root*. Leave them to infuse until tepid and use for a compress to the affected parts, applied frequently, or to sponge the skin.

• Give supplements of natural vitamin C, 200–500mg, every 2 hours to switch off the allergic reaction.

• In more chronic cases, internal treatment will be necessary, using herbs for the immune system – *camomile* and *echinacea* – with herbs for the adrenal glands – *borage*, *liquorice* or *wild yam* – combined with herbs to aid elimination via the bowels and kidneys and to clear the system, such as *burdock*, *dandelion leaves* and *root*, *fumitory*, *nettles*, *red clover* and *wild pansy*.

• As with all conditions of an allergic nature, the possibility of emotional problems should be considered, and you may want to give herbs for the nervous system, such as *camomile*, *lemon balm*, *skullcap* and *vervain*, and *Bach Flower Remedies* (see page 165).

• For more details and dietary measures see also the Immune System, page 70.

PRICKLY HEAT

This is an itchy and irritating skin condition, sometimes affecting babies and children at the onset of hot weather or when they are travelling abroad to summer climes. It develops as a rash of little red or pink spots, which are raised, resembling urticaria, and which can become blisters. They are found on exposed parts of the body, particularly the trunk, shoulders, neck and arms. The rash is made worse by sweating, so it is important to keep the child covered but cool, out of the hot sun.

Treatment of Prickly Heat

• Cool the skin by bathing the child with tepid to cool water. To this you can add infusions of *burdock*, *camomile*, *chickweed* or *marigold*.

• Prickly heat can indicate a child's inability to cope with extra heat because of excess internal heat. This can, in some cases, be related to excess 'heating' foods in the diet, poor bowel function or a congested toxic system. The removal of 'heating' foods, such as garlic, onions and spices, citrus fruits and milk produce, from the diet can often bring speedy relief.

• To cool the system, teas can be given internally. Choose from *burdock*, *camomile*, *dandelion root*, *nettles* or *peppermint*. These can be given singly or in combinations made to taste. Sweeten with *liquorice* or honey and give warm, *not hot*, three to six times daily.

SUNBURN

Babies and fair-skinned children are particularly susceptible to sunburn when they are unaccustomed to the sun, even when it is not very hot. Great care should be taken with children's delicate skin and with acclimatizing them to summer sun, especially if you are away on a holiday in the sun. A few minutes only in the sun for the first few days is plenty, and then the child should be kept lightly covered in the shade. Always keep a hat on a baby or child. The sun can be very powerful and, on a beach by the sea, it is reflected back, reaching even those sitting in the shade. Apply sun lotions liberally and frequently.

Should sunburn occur, it can cause reddening and soreness of the skin, which may be swollen and very hot. Some babies or children may develop a fever.

Treatment of Sunburn

Generally, sunburn involves first-degree burning of the skin, which can be helped considerably by herbs and natural medicines.

• First, bathe the affected skin with cold or tepid water to reduce the heat and inflammation.

• Then apply any of the following: *aloe vera gel*, *calendula ointment*, *chickweed ointment*, *comfrey juice* or *ointment*, *cucumber juice*, '*hyperical*' ointment, which is made from *hypericum* (*St John's wort*) and *calendula* (*marigold*), *lavender oil* or plain, natural yoghurt.

SKIN INFECTION

When the defence mechanisms in the skin are impaired for any reason, the skin may become infected by bacterial, fungal or viral organisms. Bacterial infections include abscesses, boils and impetigo. Viral infections include warts and verrucae and herpes. Fungal infections include athlete's foot (ringworm) and monilia (thrush).

While it is important to distinguish one condition from another and to treat it accordingly, it is also necessary to treat the child constitutionally, for only a poor skin is prone to infection. The skin reflects internal health and is related not only to a child's nutritional status, but also to the child's general level of health and emotional state. This is especially the case where there are recurrent skin infections or slow healing infections.

ABSCESSES

An abscess is a collection of pus, made up of white blood cells which have attacked bacteria invading the body, and the ensuing debris. These cells collect together, forming a boundary to block off the diseased area from the rest of the body to prevent the infection from spreading. The abscess can be small and superficial as at a finger tip, or it can develop more deeply in the body, in an internal organ. The body needs to cleanse itself of this pus, and so it discharges itself by bursting spontaneously through the surface nearest to it. The area around an abscess may be hot, swollen, red, inflamed and tender. In deep abscesses there may be fever and general malaise.

BOILS

An abscess in the skin is a boil. A pimple is a small boil. Boils are tender, red, inflamed areas, which develop from staphylococcal infection of hair follicles or sebaceous glands. As the lumps filled with pus come to the surface of the skin, they come to a head, which usually burst after a few days or spontaneously resolve themselves. They often come in crops, as bacteria can infect several surrounding hair follicles, and they tend to occur in areas of pressure – on the buttocks, in armpits, or around the neck where a collar rubs the skin, for instance – where they can be very uncomfortable and often quite painful. A carbuncle is a larger abscess, which results from the infection spreading or from several boils joining together.

Abscesses, boils and pimples should never be squeezed as this may push the discharging infection further into the skin and introduce new infection. They should be allowed to come to a head on their own, and you can encourage them to do this naturally in several ways. Consult your practitioner if a boil does not come to a head within a few days, or if red streaks spreading outwards from it appear, as this means the infection is spreading.

Repeated attacks of boils demand particular attention. They indicate impaired resistance to infection and generally run-down, congested and toxic state. This may be related to a poor diet, a sedentary life-style, excessive fatty foods and poor fat metabolism. In some cases they can be a sign of more serious illness, such as diabetes mellitus. If they do not clear with treatment, consult your practitioner.

Treatment of Abscesses and Boils

Any treatment needs to consist of external treatment to draw out the pus, combined with internal remedies to clear the hot, congested state of the tissues.

External Treatment

• Hot poultices can be applied to the area and left for an hour or so, three times daily. They can be prepared from any of the following herbs: *burdock (leaves or root)*, *chickweed*, *comfrey (leaves or root)*, *marshmallow (leaves or root)*, *nasturtium seeds*, *plantain leaves* and *slippery elm powder*. Moisten the dried herb and mash it in hot water (or mash and heat the fresh herb). Add a few drops of essential oil of *eucalyptus*, *lavender* or *thyme*. Place it on a gauze pad and apply. Cover with a clean firm bandage or dressing. Remove between applications to allow air to the area, and to stop the skin becoming too moist. Sunlight is particularly therapeutic.

• Alternatively, you could use equal parts of honey and cod liver oil on clean lint, taped or bandaged to the area. Or apply a cooked onion as a hot poultice or a paste of $\frac{1}{2}$ teaspoon

149

(2–3ml) each of *ginger* and *turmeric* powder mixed with a little water.

• Continue to apply whichever remedy you choose daily until the boil or abscess has discharged, the pain has resolved and the boil has cleared. If the boil is particularly stubborn, it may require lancing by the doctor.

Internal Treatment

Echinacea or *wild indigo* and *garlic* will help to resolve the infection and cleanse the system. Tonic herbs to help resolve heat and toxic congestion and restore vitality can be added; choose from *agrimony*, *burdock*, *nettles*, *poke root* (only in small amounts) or *red clover*. If there is constipation add *yellow dock* or *liquorice* (and follow dietary suggestions, page 138). These need to be taken in hot decoction, flavoured with *peppermint* and honey if you wish; give a cupful at least three times daily.

• Make sure that the child's diet is rich in fresh fruit and vegetables, and help the body in its cleansing efforts by avoiding excess meat, eggs, sugar, saturated fats and carbohydrates.

• You should also follow the general treatment of the immune system (see page 70).

IMPETIGO

This is a highly contagious staphylococcal infection of the skin, and it commonly affects the area around the lips, nose and ears. It starts as a rash of small blisters, which break open and become crusts and yellow-brown scabs. It is important to try to stop the child from touching weeping blisters and thus spreading the infection. Keep the child's towel or flannel or bed clothes away from those of other members of the family, and keep the child away from school until the infection clears. Impetigo can develop as a secondary infection, complicating eczema, cold sores, hives or scabies.

External Treatment of Impetigo

• Use warm decoctions of *echinacea*, *golden seal*, *marigold* or *wild indigo* to bathe the area. Pat dry gently afterwards with a paper towel.

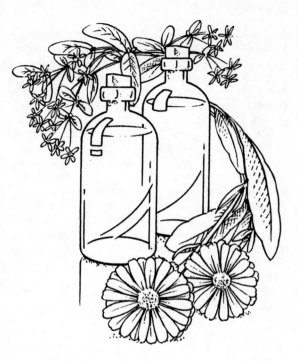

• Dilute tinctures of the above herbs can be used, and *marigold* and *St John's wort* or *myrrh* are particularly effective.

• A few drops of essential oils of *eucalyptus*, *lavender*, *tea tree* or *thyme* can be added to a bowl of hot or boiling water (or a facial steamer) and used to steam the face.

Internal Treatment of Impetigo

A decoction of equal parts of e*chinacea*, *peppermint* and *pasque flower* or *red clover*, and ½ part *poke root* can be given; a cupful three times daily.

• *Garlic* perles or honey, and supplements of vitamin C (200–500mg daily) will help the body to resolve the infection.

WARTS AND VERRUCAE

Warts are small growths made up of dead cells; they are caused by the wart virus. They can occur singly or in a number of different places anywhere on the body. When they occur on the soles of the feet they are known as verrucae, and can be painful when the child walks or stands. Warts are contagious, especially where there is moisture – such as around swimming pools and bathrooms, which is why so many children seem to catch verrucae at public swimming baths. To help prevent the spread of infection, if your child has a verruca and goes swimming, cover the foot with a special plastic sock. Always dry the feet well before getting out of the bath and put slippers on before the child steps on to the floor or the bathmat. Do not let the child run around barefoot until the verruca has gone.

Warts and verrucae often disappear spontaneously after weeks, months or even years. However, you can hasten their departure through herbal treatment.

External Treatment of Warts and Verrucae

• Several herbs can be used directly on the wart, including lemon juice, raw *garlic* clove, yellow juice from the fresh *greater celandine*, white juice from *dandelion* stalks or unripe *figs*, tincture of *thuja*, inner sides of *broad bean pods*, oil of *tea tree* and fresh *elderberry* juice. Continue until the warts disappear. This will vary from one child to another.

• If, after a few weeks, there is no sign of improvement, constitutional treatment may be necessary, paying particular attention to the immune system (see page 70).

Internal Treatment of Warts and Verrucae

Internal treatment needs to include herbs to enhance the body's vitality and its fight against the virus, as well as herbs for the liver and general cleansing of the system.

• A useful recipe, to be taken three times daily as tea or tincture, can be made from equal parts of *burdock*, *dandelion root*, *echinacea*, *kelp*, *peppermint* and *red clover*.

• *Garlic* pearles and vitamin C supplements can be taken. For dietary measures see Immune System, page 70.

HERPES AND COLD SORES

Cold sores are small blisters around the nose and lips, which usually burst and crust over before they clear up. They are caused by the herpes simplex virus which lives dormantly in nerve endings in many children after an initial infection, normally passed on by kissing an adult with the infection. It can be reactivated when the child is run down, either by other illness, such as a cold, influenza, a fever, pneumonia or poor diet or by other physical or emotional stress. It may also be related to some extent to a rise in skin temperature, as it can also be caused by sunburn and, equally, exposure to extremes of cold.

General Treatment of Cold Sores

The initial herpes infection gives rise to the blisters around the mouth, followed by painful ulcers inside the mouth and inflamed gums. These make it hard for the child to eat and drink and, in some children, there can be a fever and malaise and swollen lymph glands in the neck.

• When this occurs, treat the child normally for fever and infection (see pages 72 and 85–8), giving only liquids and nothing that requires chewing or causes smarting of the ulcers, such as sharp fruit juices.

• Try to keep the child away from close contact with other babies or children during the initial and subsequent infection, especially those with other skin problems, such as eczema or nappy rash, as these can be further complicated by secondary herpes infection.

• It is also important to discourage the child from scratching the cold sores, which can irritate or itch, as this can introduce a secondary bacterial infection such as impetigo. If this occurs, the cold sores will not clear as they should and will, instead, become red and inflamed, with pus-filled centres.

151

External Treatment of Cold Sores

• Keep a child with cold sores out of bright sunlight and make sure that you keep his or her towels and flannels separate from those used by the rest of the family.

• Avoid face contact and try and keep the hands as clean as possible in case the child touches or scratches the blisters.

• If a cold sore occurs very near the eye, consult your practitioner as it may affect the eye.

• Several herbs will help to speed healing of the blisters and discourage secondary infection: use tea or dilute tincture of *echinacea, golden seal, myrrh* or *St John's wort* mixed with *marigold*.

• Essential oils can be mixed with a little alcohol, such as tincture and then diluted with water to make an effective lotion: mix 10 drops of the oils of *lavender, oregano, tea tree* and *thyme* with 1 teaspoon (5ml) of tincture of *lavender*. Add 1 tablespoon (20ml) of water. Apply on cotton wool to the blisters three or four times a day.

• Once the infection has cleared, *comfrey ointment* can be applied twice daily to complete healing and prevent scarring. Vitamin E oil can also be applied directly to the skin.

Internal Treatment of Cold Sores

Treatment is aimed at boosting the immune system, using herbs such as *astragalus, echinacea, garlic* and *wild indigo*, as well as enhancing the elimination of toxins using alterative herbs such as *burdock, dandelion root, nettles, red clover* and *yellow dock*, with herbs to stimulate the lymphatic system, such as *cleavers, marigold* and *poke root* (only in small amounts).

• The following recipe can be used during infection and for a week or so afterwards. Mix equal parts of *peppermint, echinacea, cleavers, dandelion root* and *burdock* with $\frac{1}{2}$ part of *liquorice*.

• *Burdock* is always best taken as a tea, and it can be mixed with equal parts of *peppermint*.

Dietary Treatment of Cold Sores

(See also Immune System, page 70.)

• Supplements of natural vitamin C tablets (200–500mg morning and evening) and cod liver oil (1 teaspoon (5ml) daily) can be given.

• Some amino acids can both stimulate and inhibit activation of the virus. Lysine helps to inhibit infection by controlling multiplication of the virus; it is found in beans and bean-sprouts, brewer's yeast, chicken, lamb and in most fruits and vegetables. Arginine can help predispose to infection, and foods rich in this amino acid should be avoided if a child is prone to cold sores. These include peanuts, chocolate and carob, coconut, oats, wheat and gelatine.

RINGWORM – ATHLETE'S FOOT

This commonly affects the scalp, the feet (between the toes, when it is known as athlete's foot) and the groin, but it can affect any area of the skin, the hair or the nails. When it affects the skin on the body it gives rise to red scaly rings, which spread outwards, leaving the centre of the circular patches looking like normal skin. On the scalp it causes circular or oval patches which as they spread, leave a centre of healed skin, but also of broken-off hairs, causing patches of baldness. When it occurs between the toes it is red and inflamed and can cause not only intense itching, as it can elsewhere, but also cracking of the skin between the toes, which can make it painful.

Ringworm is highly contagious and is often contracted from infected pets or farm animals. Warm, moist conditions are ideal for the growth and spread of the infection, such as in swimming pools, bathrooms or changing rooms, or sweating. It is often extremely resilient to treatment, especially when it arises as athlete's foot and it is immune to most disinfectants. To prevent the spread of the infection within the family use separate towels and hair brushes, and wash hands thoroughly after touching infected areas. Check your pets for infection, as they may need treating too.

Internal Treatment of Ringworm

Herbs can be taken to boost immunity, raise vitality and encourage elimination.

● Use the equal parts of *cleavers, dandelion root, echinacea, nettles, peppermint* and *red clover*, and give *burdock* and *peppermint* tea. *Garlic* perles should be taken daily.

External Treatment of Ringworm

You may want to try a variety of different remedies to find which is best for your family.

● You can seal the infected area off from air to inhibit the infection, by painting on either undiluted lemon juice or egg white repeatedly to form a glaze several times a day.

● Undiluted oils of *lavender, lemon, oregano, tea tree* or *thyme* can be applied three times daily with cotton wool.

● Tinctures of *blood root, echinacea, golden seal, iodine, marigold, myrrh* or *thuja* can be applied singly or in mixtures, three times daily.

● A crushed *garlic* clove can be rubbed into the area.

● Bathe the feet in decoctions or infusions of *agrimony, blood root, burdock, golden seal, marigold* or *poke root*. Make sure that the area is always dried well, especially between and underneath the toes.

PARASITIC INFECTIONS OF THE SKIN

SCABIES

This is an intensely itchy skin condition caused by a tiny female mite, which burrows into the skin and lays eggs. It can occur anywhere but is commonly found in between the fingers, on the hands and wrists, the elbows and armpits, genitals and feet. There is a rash of small blisters and tiny lines where the marks are made in the skin by the mites burrowing; the lines are the main diagnostic guide to the con-

dition. Some children develop an allergy to the mites, which causes urticaria (see page 147). The itching is made worse by warmth, so is often very annoying when in bed.

Scabies are highly contagious. When the eggs hatch they are passed from one person to another by direct contact (and so can be found on the trunk of a baby who has been picked up by an infected parent) or from bed linen, clothing (where it can survive for about two weeks) or from pets.

To discourage the spread of infection keep clothing, bedding and towels separate and have your pets treated by the vet. Try to discourage a child from scratching, as this may introduce a secondary infection into the skin. Keep the hands as clean as possible by washing them frequently.

Treatment of Scabies

Scabies can be difficult to eradicate, especially since it takes from six to eight weeks for the symptoms of intense itching to appear. It is best to treat all the family at the same time to avoid confusion.

● A long hot bath should be given at night, and then the skin should be dried briskly, to open up the pores and the burrows.

● Then apply dilute oils of *bergamot, lavender, peppermint, rosemary* or *tea tree*, or an infusion or decoction or a dilute tincture of *echinacea, golden seal, poke root* or *tansy* over the whole body.

● Put on clean nightclothes and get into clean bedclothes.

● Repeat the process on the following two nights.

● Some itching may occur for the next few days, but this does not mean that the infection is not clearing.

● Take the following remedy *internally*. Mix equal parts of *cleavers, dandelion root, echinacea, peppermint* and *red clover*, and give *garlic perles* daily.

● Wash all clothing, towels and bed linen

thoroughly on a hot wash and iron afterwards when dry. Leave for three weeks before using them again.

HEAD LICE

Three types of louse can affect our bodies: the head louse, the body louse and the pubic (or crab) louse. The latter two predominantly affect adults. Head lice are epidemic in school-age children, and they are fast becoming 'super lice' as they become immune to treatment. They move from one child to another by close contact, especially from long hair, which is not tied up, and they can live for twenty-four hours away from the body. They are pale greyish-brown and are hard to see; they are most easily found at the back of the head, hiding in the hair. The female louse lays approximately eight eggs a day, which stick to the hair and are visible as little white specks; these are called nits. After eight days the eggs hatch, and each louse lives for a further five weeks or so, piercing the skin on the scalp several times a day when hungry to feed from the blood, and causing the characteristic itching and scratching of the scalp. The bites produce inflammation of the skin, which looks like red pinpricks on the scalp.

If there is severe infestation of the head, the inflammation on the scalp can lead to infection, introduced through scratching, and the child may have swollen neck glands.

Treatment of Head Lice

Head lice can be treated effectively using essential oils in a base of olive oil, which needs to be rubbed into the hair and scalp at night and left on until morning when it should be washed out thoroughly. The child should sleep on a towel to prevent the bedclothes becoming stained with oil. When the hair is covered in oil, use a nit-comb to remove the nits. They can be difficult to shift as they can stick hard to the shaft of the hair. Dipping the comb in hot vinegar will help to loosen them.

Recipe for Treating Head Lice

25 drops lavender oil
10 drops geranium oil
25 drops rosemary oil
1 dessertspoon (12ml) eucalyptus oil
2 teaspoons (10ml) tea tree oil

Mix the ingredients in 4fl oz (100ml) base oil (olive, almond or sunflower). Apply each night for five nights, then repeat for two nights after a week – and your problems should be solved! Make sure you keep hairbrushes and towels separate from other members of the family.

THE URINARY SYSTEM

The urinary system performs the vital task of producing and excreting urine, so cleansing the body of waste products and helping to maintain

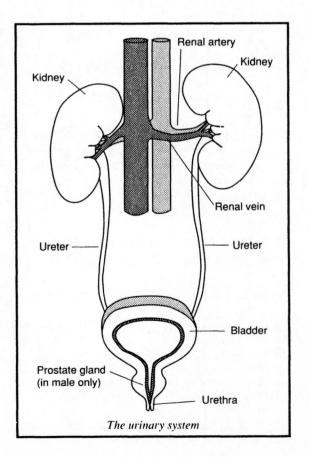

The urinary system

a constant internal environment by governing the water and chemical composition and the acid/alkali balance of the body. It is important to encourage a child to drink plenty each day to assist the kidneys in their cleansing work, to flush through toxins and waste products of metabolism and to prevent them from causing irritation of the urinary tract along the way.

During any kind of infection or inflammatory process, you can help the body to throw off accumulated toxins and any debris produced in the system from the immune system's battle against infection and inflammation (see Immune System, page 61), by using diuretic herbs, which increase the flow of urine. These herbs include *buchu, celery seed, cleavers, corn silk, couch grass, dandelion leaf, juniper* and *uva ursi*.

URINARY TRACT INFECTIONS

Urinary tract infections can occur quite commonly in children. They affect about 3 per cent of boys and 5 per cent of girls at some time before puberty. Infections in babies can be due to structural abnormalities, but they are most frequently caused by bacteria from the bowel (*E. coli*) affecting the bladder. They creep round from the anus, helped by wiping from back to front rather than vice-versa after urination or a bowel movement. They affect girls more than boys because of the difference in their anatomy; the urinary passage (urethra) to the bladder is much shorter in girls. Vaginal infections such as thrush can also be related to urinary tract infections.

Infection can affect the urethra, then pass into the bladder, causing cystitis. From the bladder it can pass along the ureters to affect the kidneys (pyelonephritis). Other kidney infections (nephritis) can develop as secondaries from other childhood infections, such as a streptococcal throat infection causing tonsilitis.

A urinary infection may be low grade and cause few symptoms, or it may occur in a child who is too young to tell you how they feel, so it may be hard to diagnose in some children, except by urine analysis. More commonly, however, it produces the symptoms listed in the box below.

Treatment of Urinary Tract Infections

• If your child develops a urinary tract infection, use soothing diuretics to relieve the burning or pain when passing water, such as *comfrey, corn silk, couch grass* and *marshmallow*.

• Combine these with anti-inflammatory, antiseptic herbs for the urinary tract, such as *buchu, camomile, horsetail, uva ursi* and *yarrow*.

• A useful prescription, which can be very effective, is made from equal parts of *buchu, camomile, couch grass, horsetail* and *uva ursi*.

• Infusions should be left to infuse for 10–20 minutes and then taken luke-warm to cold every hour or two through the day. They can also be used for hand and foot baths, and in a bowl for a shallow bath – the child can sit in this for 10 minutes twice a day.

• If there is fever and backache or lower abdominal pain, you should suspect a kidney infection, *in which case call your practitioner*. Use the above herbs and add herbs for fever management such as *boneset, camomile, elderflowers, limeflowers* and *yarrow*, and use these for teas (taken frequently through the day), and for tepid sponging and hand and foot baths.

• Make sure your child drinks plenty through the day. Herbal teas can be alternated with soothing barley water.

Barley Water

Simmer 4oz (100g) of washed barley in 1 pint (600ml) of water until the barley is soft. Add a little lemon and honey and drink luke-warm, several times daily.

Symptoms of Urinary Infection

☐ An urge to pass water frequently
☐ Urgency to pass water
☐ Bed-wetting
☐ Strong smelling, cloudy urine
☐ Pain or crying on passing water
☐ Fever and malaise
☐ Lower back ache or abdominal pain
☐ Vomiting
☐ Headache

● Give regular drinks of *cranberry juice* to counteract the infection. You can also add a little baking soda to a glass of water – ½ teaspoon (2–3ml) to a glass of water – to alkalize the urine.

If your child is prone to recurrent urinary infections, consult your doctor as it may be due to an anatomical problem. Alternatively, it can be related to food allergy (see Immune System, page 61).

BED-WETTING

Most children become potty trained in the daytime some time before they can go through the night without wetting the bed. Very often the child can be kept in nappies at night until he or she is dry regularly in the morning or the child decides he or she does not want them on any more. A potty by the side of the bed will make it much easier for a small child to pass water in the night without waking up the rest of the house – leave a dim light on in the bedroom so that he or she can see.

If a child sleeps particularly heavily it may take longer for him or her to be dry at night than others, but most children go through the night without wetting the bed when they are two or three years old.

Causes of Bed-wetting

Bed-wetting that occurs in a child older than four or five years who has already developed bladder control is frequently related to stress. It could be jealousy of a new baby, anxiety about moving house, changing school, trouble with school work, teachers, peers, upset over family rows or anything else that causes stress, over-excitement, insecurity or unhappiness. If this is the case your child will need plenty of love and reassurance from you, and not reprimanding for something that cannot be helped. It can be quite humiliating for an older child to find that he or she has wet the bed and that other people know about it.

● If your child has never been dry regularly at night, it may be that the nerves and muscles governing bladder function are not yet mature enough.

● Once a child is over four years and still wetting the bed regularly, it is worth getting a medical check to ascertain whether there is any

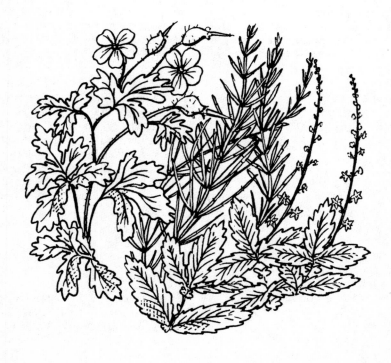

underlying physical condition causing bed-wetting. Possible causes include diabetes, a hidden urinary infection, a structural abnormality of the urinary system, dietary deficiencies (particularly of calcium and magnesium), over-use of refined foods and sugar, over-sensitivity to food additives or chemicals in drinking water or a food allergy.

• Some children tend to wet the bed more if they get cold, so make sure they are always well covered, and put extra clothes on if they habitually kick the bedclothes off at night.

Treatment of Bed-wetting

• Avoid giving too much to drink before bed, and give teas of *St John's wort*, *horsetail* and *corn silk* through the day, and a little before bed, sweetened with honey, to soothe an irritated bladder and to encourage normal nervous control of the bladder.

• Other useful remedies include *agrimony*, *American cranesbill*, *herb Robert* and *parsley*.

• If you feel your child's bed-wetting stems from emotional disturbance, add *lemon balm*, *skullcap*, *vervain* or *wild oats* to the remedy, to relax and soothe the nerves.

• Massage oil of *camomile* or *St John's wort* into the lower spine and abdomen while settling the child down for sleep.

• Always reward your child for a dry bed – and this will actively encourage him or her to stop wetting it – and do not let your child think that it is a problem that you are worrying about.

• *Bach Flower Remedies – mimulus, aspen, star of Bethlehem* or *sweet chestnut* – may be helpful (see page 165).

FEBRILE CONVULSIONS

A convulsion is a fit or seizure caused by an abnormal burst of electrical activity in the brain. It involves a sudden muscular spasm,

when the child may become rigid for a few seconds while holding the breath, and then has repeated jerky movements of the arms and legs or the whole body. He or she may cry out as the fit starts, and may pass urine or a stool, and then fall unconscious. After this the child will want to sleep, during which time recovery will occur. Some children have very mild fits, when the eyes turn upwards and the body goes stiff for just a few seconds.

Convulsions can be very frightening, both for the child and the parents, but normally, if you just make sure the child does not hurt him or herself by jerky limb movements, no harm will come from them.

Causes of Convulsions

Luckily, fits are not that common in babies or children. They can occur with or without fevers.

• The most common cause of a convulsion or fit is a high fever, especially in babies and children up to the age of three years. These febrile convulsions are not often seen in a child older than five years. They can be related to any childhood infection that is characterized by a high fever, and the Chinese say that they are more likely when an infection involves a lot of phlegm or catarrh in the system.

• Your child may be prone to convulsions if there is a family history of convulsions, in which case they can occur with any change of temperature, not necessarily a very high fever.

• If fits occur frequently in a child, you will become quite accustomed to dealing with them and they will be less threatening. Some children prone to convulsions are given anti-convulsive drugs during infections for fear that frequent or long fits will cause brain damage. However, most children who have a febrile convulsion once never have another one.

Treatment of Convulsions

To prevent febrile convulsions it is important to keep an eye on all fevers in children. If the temperature rises above 102°F (38.8°C) you can lower it by giving herbs to increase

THE HERBAL FOR MOTHER AND CHILD

perspiration and resolve fever (see Fever Management, page 85–8) and by tepid sponging using these infusions, until the temperature is down to 100°F (38°C).

• It is also important to keep an unwell child with a fever quiet and resting and, when the child is distressed, to soothe them using herbs, and massage or *Bach Flower Remedies* and your comforting presence to calm him or her.

• When your child has a fever, include *catmint, limeflowers, skullcap* or *valerian* in your prescription, and use these also for tepid sponging, and hand and foot baths.

• Teas of *cardamon* and *dill seeds* or *peppermint* can also be helpful.

• Give *Bach Flower Remedies* – *Rescue Remedy, rock rose, mimulus* or *aspen* (see page 165).

• Massage the child with dilute oils of *camomile, lavender, melissa* or *ylang ylang* to help keep him or her calm and relaxed.

• If your baby or child has a convulsion hold him or her over your knee to ensure that the tongue does not fall backwards and obstruct the airway. Do not try to put anything in the mouth or restrict the movements.

• Once the fit is over, lie the child on his or her side to sleep so that the tongue or saliva are not inhaled. Drop a little *Star of Bethlehem* (Bach Flower Remedy) on the temples or wrists.

Call your doctor if your baby or child has a fit as the cause may need to be investigated. It could be due to epilepsy or meningitis. If your baby has had a fit, your doctor will advise against giving a whooping cough vaccination and, possibly, the measles vaccine.

CHAPTER 10

INFECTIOUS CHILDHOOD DISEASES

CHICKEN POX

This is a viral infection that is spread easily among children, particularly those under ten years of age, by contact and droplets of saliva spread through talking, coughing or sneezing. A child is most infectious just before the spots come out, and remains so until all the blisters have dried up, which takes about a week. The incubation period is seventeen to twenty-one days.

It starts with a headache, a fever and general malaise. There may be swollen lymph glands. The spots start normally on the trunk and can appear on the face, the scalp, inside the mouth, anus, vagina or ears; the arms and legs tend to be the least affected. They appear in crops every three or four days, starting as little pimples and quickly developing into oval-shaped blisters, which are filled with fluid. Gradually the spots dry up and scab over. The scabs fall off after about ten days, and may leave scars, some of which are permanent, especially if the spots have been scratched.

The blisters can be very itchy, and it is important to discourage your child from scratching as much as you can. Not only does scratching leave scars, but it also introduces bacterial infection into the skin, which can lead to impetigo, conjunctivitis or boils.

Symptoms of Chicken Pox

- ☐ Headache
- ☐ Fever, usually mild
- ☐ Malaise
- ☐ Swollen lymph nodes
- ☐ Blotchy rash, which disappears as the blisters appear
- ☐ Red pimples, which develop into itchy oval blisters
- ☐ Blisters are filled with clear fluid; this turns cloudy and then dries up
- ☐ The spots scab over, and the scabs fall off

Rarely, chicken pox can lead to encephalitis or be complicated by Reye's Syndrome. If your child feels unwell again once the scabs have healed and has a headache, vomits or feels particularly drowsy, call your doctor immediately.

If your child has blisters on the eyeball call your doctor.

The chicken pox virus is related to the one that causes shingles, and a child may catch chicken pox from an adult with shingles, but rarely vice versa. If you are pregnant and have been in contact with chicken pox and are not immune, contact your doctor.

Treatment of Chicken Pox

• As with all infectious diseases, you can speed recovery through treating the immune system by using *garlic* and *echinacea*.

• Very often a child feels only mildly unwell, but if there is a fever add *boneset*, *camomile* and *yarrow*. You can use the following recipe. Equal parts of *boneset*, *camomile*, *echinacea* and *yarrow* and give as a warm tea, sweetened with honey or blackcurrant juice if you wish. Give ½ a cup every two hours.

• If your child feels unwell, restless or uncomfortable, add *camomile*, *catnip* or *skullcap*.

• To help clear the skin quickly and relieve the itching, give tea of *burdock*, *camomile*, *elderflowers* and *heartsease* frequently through the day.

• Externally, to help relieve the itching and speed healing of the skin, wash the skin frequently with any of the following: *camomile*, *chickweed*, *lavender*, *marigold*, *raspberry leaves* or *St John's wort*.

Use cool infusions and apply them on cotton wool or a flannel, or add them to bath water.

- Distilled *witch hazel* can be diluted and applied; it may feel extra good when ice-cold.

- Decoctions of *burdock*, *golden seal* or *yellow dock* can be sponged on to the spots to relieve severe itching. Rub dry and then pat the skin with a little *arrowroot*.

- Essential oils of *camomile*, *lavender*, *peppermint* or *tea tree* can be dropped into water and applied as compresses, or used in bath water.

- If spots become infected, bathe them frequently with *golden seal* or *marigold*, or dilute *tea tree oil*. Clean them with dilute *witch hazel*.

- Once the blisters have dried and the scabs have fallen off, use *comfrey ointment*, alternated with dilute *lavender oil*, to prevent scar formation and to heal the skin properly. *Marigold cream* or oil and *St John's wort oil* are also beneficial.

- If there are painful blisters in the mouth, swab or give the child tea or dilute tincture of *marigold* or *golden seal* to wash the mouth with.

- If a baby has spots on the bottom, leave the nappy off as much as possible. Cut the fingernails to help stop infection.

- Give only a light diet, with mostly fruit, vegetables and soups, and plenty to drink.

MUMPS

This is caused by a viral infection that affects the salivary and parotid glands, in front of and beneath the ears. It rarely occurs in children under two years of age, and it takes two or three weeks to incubate. It is infectious for a day before the glands swell up until three days after they have gone down.

Your child will feel unwell, seem off colour and often irritable for a day or two. Then a fever may develop with a headache and pains around the neck. Then the face swells up, often first one side then the other, sometimes so much that the whole face and chin look swollen. The swelling may cause pain on swallowing and a dry mouth, and eating and talking may be very uncomfortable. Sharp or acid foods, such as lemon juice, may cause pain as

they stimulate the inflamed salivary glands.

The swelling takes from three to seven days to go down, and during that time your child will probably only feel mildly unwell. Some behave as if they are completely well. If it occurs in teenage boys or men it can cause inflammation of the testes (orchitis), and in older girls it can inflame the ovaries and cause abdominal pain. Rarely, it can lead to pancreatitis.

If, after ten days, your child develops a severe headache or a stiff neck, call your doctor immediately, as it may mean meningitis or encephalitis.

Treatment of Mumps

- To help resolve infection and fever, give *garlic* and *echinacea*, combined with *boneset*, *yarrow*, *limeflowers*, *peppermint*, *elderflowers* or *camomile*. Sweeten with honey or blackcurrant juice, or flavour with *liquorice*.

- Add *red clover*, *cleavers*, *marigold* and a little *poke root* to help reduce the congestion and swelling of the glands.

- A useful recipe you can use is:

1 part *echinacea*   1 part *cleavers*
1 part *boneset* $\frac{1}{4}$ part *poke root*
1 part *yarrow*
1 part *elderflowers*

Make an infusion or give in tincture form (10 drops in a little water or juice) every two hours.

- Massage the neck gently with dilute oils of *camomile*, *eucalyptus*, *lavender* or *thyme*, and use these for steam inhalations and for the bath. These can also be used for warm compresses.

- You could try other warm compresses using $\frac{1}{2}$ teaspoon (2–3ml) of *cayenne* powder in a cup of vinegar, or 3 parts of *mullein* to 1 part of *lobelia*, or equal parts of *poke root*, *red clover*, *marigold* and *cleavers*. Replace the compress every 30 minutes, and leave one on overnight, to help reduce the swelling and discomfort in the glands.

- You may need to liquidize foods, but give

plenty of fruit and vegetable juices – feed them through a straw if necessary.

● You can make fruit jellies from fruit juice and *agar agar* or *Iceland moss*.

● Give drinks frequently through the day, and use dilute teas of *red clover*, *marigold*, *thyme* or *cleavers* to wash the mouth out when it feels very dry and uncomfortable.

● A hot-water bottle against the painful side may alleviate some of the pain. Try wrapping the cloth you have soaked in mixtures for compresses around the hot-water bottle.

● Tepid sponge the child if the fever gets high, using infusions of *camomile*, *marigold*, *red clover*, *thyme* or *yarrow*.

MEASLES

This is a viral infection that is highly contagious and for this reason it tends to occur in epidemics. It starts like an ordinary cold, with a runny nose or a dry cough, and then a slight fever develops, often conjunctivitis, a cough and a cold. There may be the characteristic koplik's spots in the mouth – white spots on the lining of the cheeks. The fever tends to get increasingly high, often to 105°F (40°C) as the rash comes out on the third or fourth day. Flat, brownish-red spots start, usually behind the ears, and on the face and neck. They then spread to the body – less so to the arms and legs – and merge together to form red patches. Once the rash has come out properly, the fever should subside and the child will begin to feel better. As the rash starts and the fever is high, a child will feel unwell, with little or no appetite, swollen lymph nodes in the neck, often diarrhoea, vomiting and abdominal pains. There can also be earache. Measles spots do not itch. Measles is spread by droplet infection from saliva sprayed when talking, coughing or sneezing. The incubation period is between eight and fourteen days from exposure, but a child may be infectious seven days after being infected until ten days after the rash begins. Children who have been immunized may only get the respiratory symptoms of a cold or cough, *but they are still contagious*. This makes diagnosis and isolation from those babies and

Symptoms of Measles
☐ Runny nose or a cough
☐ Slight fever, rising sharply over the next few days
☐ Headache
☐ Red, sore eyes (conjunctivitis)
☐ Koplik's spots in the mouth
☐ Rash on the third or fourth day, starting behind the ears, face and neck
☐ Rash (not itchy) spreads over face and body
☐ Fever should start to subside once the rash is out
☐ Little or no appetite
☐ Swollen lymph nodes in the neck; possibly earache
☐ Diarrhoea/vomiting/abdominal pain

children who are not immunized very difficult. If there is a measles epidemic around and your immunized child develops cold symptoms, it is best to keep them away from other children.

In some children complications can occur. Pneumonia, middle ear infection and bronchitis are the most usual complications. More rarely, encephalitis can occur. Keep a close eye on a child who is recovering from measles. By the seventh or ninth day of the illness the child should be feeling better. If the temperature rises again or your child seems unwell, call your doctor.

See also Middle Ear Infection, p. 102, Pneumonia, p. 108, and Bronchitis, p. 107.

Treatment of Measles

As in all other infectious diseases with a fever, you need to support the body's efforts in throwing off the illness, which will help the body to resolve the infection quickly and without complications.

● To enhance the immune system give *garlic* and *echinacea*, combined with herbs to encourage perspiration and help resolve the fever. Choose from *boneset*, *camomile*, *catnip*, *elderflowers*, *limeflowers*, *peppermint* and *yarrow*.

● For tepid sponging, and adding to bath

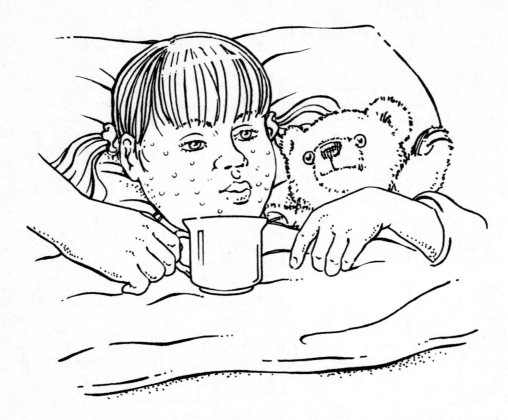

water, or hand and foot baths use *camomile,
echinacea, elderflowers, marigold, marshmallow,
red clover* or *yarrow,* or use esssential oils of
camomile, eucalyptus or *lavender* diluted in
water. These can also be used in vaporizers and
room sprays.

• At the first stage of the illness, before the
rash comes out, you can use compresses of
ginger or *thyme* applied to the skin, to help
bring out the toxins and speed it on its way.
Burdock and *peppermint* tea should be given
internally every two hours until the rash comes
out and then subsides.

• For sore, inflamed eyes use infusions made
from boiled or distilled water with *camomile,
elderflowers, eyebright* or *marigold* to bathe the
eyes. Use cotton wool and apply the tea, using a
new piece for each eye.

• If the child is irritable or restless, and has
trouble getting comfortable give plenty of

camomile or *catnip* tea. If the child is unhappy
and clingy, add *pasque flower* to the mixture.

• Make sure your child drinks plenty,
especially if the fever is high, to avoid dehydration.

• Give no solid food, just fruit and vegetable
juices or soups, until the fever has gone and the
child feels a bit better.

• Give supplements of *garlic perles* and
vitamin C.

GERMAN MEASLES (Rubella)

German measles is a viral infection, but it is
often so mild that you may not even realize
your child has had it.

It usually starts with a runny nose, loss of
appetite, sometimes a sore throat, swelling and
tenderness of the lymph nodes at the back of
the neck and behind the ears. About a day later,

a rash appears behind the ears and on the fore-head, and then spreads over the body. The rash consists of flat, small, pink spots, which may be dense enough to make the skin look red. The skin is itchy but generally recovers within three days. There may be a low-grade fever or none at all, and your child will seem fairly well.

German measles is very contagious, and has an incubation period of two or three weeks. Although the symptoms it causes in children are mild, the infection can have serious impli-cations for the unborn baby if a pregnant woman becomes infected. It can cause miscar-riage or congenital problems including deaf-ness, eye problems and heart deformities. It is wise for any woman of child-bearing age to have blood tests to check whether she has immunity to German measles. If not, she can be vaccinated. Most girls are immunized rou-tinely when they are small or at the age of twelve. If a woman has had the infection or a vaccination she should not become pregnant for another two months.

If you know your child has been in contact with German measles, it is sensible to keep them at home while they are contagious, which will be from seven days before the rash comes out. Be especially careful to keep them away from any pregnant woman.

Treatment of German Measles

The symptoms of German measles are usually so mild that no treatment may be necessary.

● If a fever develops, give teas of *camomile*, *elderflowers*, *limeflowers*, *peppermint* or *yarrow*.

● Add *marigold* or *cleavers* for the lymphatic system, and *echinacea* to enhance the efforts of the immune system.

● Externally, you can massage dilute oils of *lavender*, *thyme* or *rosemary* into the swollen lymph glands to help resolve the infection.

● If the skin is itchy and your child seems irritable, you can bathe the skin with teas of *burdock*, *camomile*, *chickweed*, *lavender*, *marsh-mallow* or *yarrow*.

● Distilled *witch hazel* or rose water are also effective.

GLANDULAR FEVER

Glandular fever or infectious mononucleosis is a viral infection. It starts with influenza-like symptoms – aches and pains, tiredness and malaise, a runny nose, sore throat and fever and sometimes a rash resembling German measles. It affects teenagers more than any other age group, but children can catch it, although they tend to be less ill with it. The main characteris-tic of glandular fever is the swollen lymph glands, most commonly occurring in the neck, and the tiredness and lethargy that the illness tends to leave in its wake, often for several weeks or months afterwards. The spleen may also be enlarged, although this causes no symp-toms.

For a clear diagnosis of glandular fever, a blood test can be carried out while the virus is active. During the post-viral period the test may not prove positive. The virus can recur, so be watchful for any symptoms that could indi-cate this and treat them promptly to minimize the risk of a long post-viral period of fatigue.

Treatment of Glandular Fever

The sooner this infection is treated, the less the debilitating effect that it will have and the quicker your child will be back to normal.

● For fever, use teas of *boneset*, *camomile*, *elderflowers*, *limeflowers*, *peppermint* or *yarrow* (see also Fever Management, page 85–8). Give the teas frequently throughout the day, alter-nated with hot lemon and honey and unswee-tened blackcurrant drinks.

● The same herbal teas can be used for tepid sponging if necessary, as well as in hand and foot baths.

● Add remedies specifically for the lymphatic system such as *cleavers*, *marigold* and small amounts of *poke root*, and *echinacea* for the immune system.

● *Garlic*, vitamin C and cod liver oil supple-ments will also be helpful (see Immune System, page 70).

● Hand and foot baths using the following herbs should be given night and morning:

calendula, *echinacea*, *golden seal*, *myrrh*, *poke root* and *wormwood*. Bathe hands for 8 minutes in the morning and the feet for 8 minutes in the evening until the child is better.

● Massage swollen lymph glands with dilute oils of *eucalyptus*, *lavender*, *pine*, *rosemary*, *rosewood* or *thyme*, or apply hot compresses of *cleavers*, *marigold* or *poke root*, mixing the infusion with a little *ginger*.

● Once the acute symptoms have subsided and the glands are less swollen, keep your child as quiet as possible and persuade him or her to rest frequently and not to try to rush back into normal activities too soon.

● For convalescence use equal parts of *dandelion root*, *echinacea*, *ginger*, *marigold*, *nettles* and *vervain*, sweetened with *liquorice* or honey, or unsweetened blackcurrant juice if you like. Give four times daily.

CONVALESCENCE AFTER INFECTIONS

To aid convalescence after infections the following recipes could be used;

Blackberry Syrup

Place 1lb (500g) blackberries and 3 tablespoons (60ml) water with 8oz (250g) sugar in a bain-marie or in a covered bowl placed in a saucepan of water. Bring the water to the boil and simmer for two hours. Strain and press the liquid through muslin into a saucepan. Add 8oz (250g) sugar and heat slowly until the sugar is dissolved. Boil hard for 5 minutes. Skim, cool and pour into bottles with screw tops or corks. This keeps in a refrigerator for several months. Dilute with cold or hot water, add a little lemon if you like. It tastes delicious.

Borage Flower Syrup

Pour sufficient boiling water over two handfuls of fresh borage flowers to cover them, in a bowl or teapot; cover and leave them to infuse overnight. Strain. Bring the liquid to the boil and pour over another two handfuls of fresh borage flowers. Cover and leave to infuse overnight again. Strain. Measure the liquid and add an equal quantity of brown sugar. Heat slowly until the sugar is dissolved, then boil fast for 5 minutes. Skim. When it is cool, pour into a bottle with a screw-on cap or cork. Store in a cool dark place. Adults should take 1–2 dessertspoons (20–40ml); children should take 1 dessertspoonful (15ml) twice daily.

Nettle Soup

1lb (500g) nettle tops
$\frac{1}{2}$oz (15g) butter
1 small onion
$\frac{1}{2}$oz (15g) flour
$\frac{3}{4}$ pint (450ml) water or stock
$\frac{1}{4}$ pint (150ml) milk
nutmeg
lemon juice
salt and pepper

Wash the nettle tops (use only young nettles) and cook them for 15 minutes in boiling, salted water. Strain but keep the water. Melt the butter in a pan, add finely chopped onion and fry until soft. Stir in the flour, add the water and boil until the liquid is thickened, stirring all the time. Add the nettles and cook gently for 15 minutes. Liquidize and return to the pan. Stir in the milk and add grated nutmeg, the lemon juice and season with salt and pepper.

Other remedies include *agrimony*, *borage*, *burdock*, *dandelion root*, *lemon balm*, *nettles* (see the recipe for nettle soup above), *red clover* and *vervain*. These should be taken three times daily in infusions after a debilitating illness or during a long winter when the body's natural defences have been weakened.

Add *chickweed* and young *dandelion* leaves to salads. *Slippery elm food*, which is easily digested, soothing and nutritious, is excellent for use in convalescence.

APPENDIX 1

THE BACH FLOWER REMEDIES

The Bach Flower Remedies are prepared from the flowers of wild plants, bushes and trees and are aimed at helping to resolve emotional and psychological disturbances, which are at the root of many physical imbalances.

For Fear

Rock Rose – for fright, panic, terror, hysteria. A remedy for emergencies, even when there appears no hope.

Mimulus – for fear of everyday known things, such as illness, death, old age, pain, darkness or being alone. Also for shyness and fear of other people. These fears are kept inside and are not spoken of to others.

Cherry Plum – fear of being overstrained or losing control over body, mind or emotions, such as uncontrollable anger and other impulses which may cause harm to oneself or others; including suicidal tendencies.

Aspen – for vague, unknown fears, a sense of foreboding, nightmares or terror of approaching misfortune for no apparent reason. One is often afraid to talk about these fears to other people.

Red Chestnut – for overconcern or fear about the welfare of others, especially loved ones, during time such as illness, journeys, when away from one's side. Often one does not worry for oneself.

For Uncertainty

Cerato – for doubt about one's ability to make decisions and judgements, and for constantly seeking advice from others and often being misguided.

Scleranthus – for indecision, inability to choose between two things, changing one's mind; energy and mood swings. For people

who are quiet and tend not to talk about their difficulties to others.

Gentian – for people who are easily discouraged, in whom small set-backs can cause depression, despondency or self-doubt, even though generally they are doing well.

Gorse – for great hopelessness, feelings of despair and futility. For giving up believing that any more can be done for them. If pushed or to please others, they may try various treatments with little real hope of improvement.

Hornbeam – for those who feel they need strengthening and help physically or mentally to bear the burden life has placed upon their shoulders. For 'Monday-morning' feeling, not feeling up to facing the coming day, the pressures of everyday life.

Wild Oat – for those who feel dissatisfied in their way of life, but have difficulty in determining what path to follow, though their ambition is strong.

For Insufficient Interest in Present Circumstances

Clematis – for people who have a tendency to daydream, think about the future, and do not live fully in the present. For lack of concentration, making little effort in everyday life, and for living in hope of happier times ahead.

Honeysuckle – for those who live in the past, and do not expect happiness as they have enjoyed before. For nostalgia, homesickness, reminiscing.

Wild Rose – for those who resign themselves to their present circumstances, and make little effort to find joy or happiness. For uncomplaining apathy.

Olive – for complete mental and physical

exhaustion. Daily life seems hard, without joy and wearisome. Those people are worn out from mental or physical ordeals and suffering.

White Chestnut – for persistent unwanted thoughts and ideas which, though thrown out, return when there is not sufficient interest in the present to fully occupy the mind. For mental arguments, preoccupations, obsessive thoughts which cause mental torture, and an inability to relax or concentrate fully on work or leisure in the day.

Mustard – for periods of sadness, gloom or even despair, which descends for no apparent reason, making it impossible to feel happiness or joy.

Chestnut Bud – for those who do not learn from observation and experience and constantly repeat the same experiences and make the same mistakes, before their lesson is learnt.

For Loneliness

Water Violet – for very quiet people who appear aloof, and prefer to be alone. They are independent and self-reliant, often bright and talented, and do not tend to get involved in other people's affairs. They radiate peace and tranquility to those around them.

Impatiens – for those who think and act quickly, and so want everything done without delay. They are often happier working or being alone so that they can go at their own speed, for they are often impatient or irritated by others who do things more slowly.

Heather – for people who need to discuss their affairs with other people and so seek the company of anybody who will listen. They become very unhappy if they are left alone for any length of time.

For Being Oversensitive to Ideas and Influences

Agrimony – for cheerful, jovial people who hide their troubles behind their humour, not wishing to burden others with them. They will go to great lengths to avoid arguments or disharmony, and may use alcohol or drugs to stimulate them and help them cope cheerfully with their pain or anxiety.

Centaury – for kind people who find it hard to say 'no', being over-anxious to please and serve others and tending to work harder on other people's behalf than on their own particular calling or interests. They are easily exploited.

Walnut – for breaking links with the past and helping adjustments to new phases (such as new relationships, jobs, houses), balancing emotions in transition periods (such as starting school, puberty, marriage, menopause) or even death of a loved one. The remedy helps protect one from outside influences which may cause one to stray from a chosen path.

Holly – for people who are overcome by negative emotions such as anger, jealousy, envy and suspicion. They suffer much inside, often when there is no real cause.

For Despondency or Despair

Larch – for people who do not consider themselves as good or as capable as those around them. Even though they may be perfectly able, they lack confidence and expect failure, so that often they do not try hard enough to succeed: the self-fulfilling prophecy.

Pine – for people who blame themselves and feel guilty. Even when they succeed, they are not satisfied with their efforts or results, and feel they could have done better. They work hard and suffer much from the faults they attach to themselves, even claiming responsibility for mistakes which are not theirs.

Elm – for diligent people, who are doing good work, often helping others, and following a vocation, but who feel overburdened or overextended at times, which causes depression or despondency.

Sweet Chestnut – for those who feel that the anguish is so great it is unbearable, they have reached the limits of their endurance, and there is nothing left but dark despair.

Star of Bethlehem – for great distress and unhappiness following some kind of shock, such as bad news, the death of a loved one or an accident.

Willow – for those who feel bitter or resentful about their misfortune, and, as a result, take less interest in the things in life they used to enjoy doing. They feel that life is injust and unfair.

Oak – for those who never give up, despite setbacks, misfortune or illness. They keep trying one thing after another, determined to reach their goal. Never losing hope, they fight on.

Crab Apple – for cleansing. For people who feel self-disgust or contamination, feelings of shame or low self-esteem. Concentrating obsessively on one shameful aspect of themselves and ignoring others. For detoxification of the body, and cleansing of wounds, whether emotional or physical, internal or external.

For Overconcern with the Welfare of Others

Chicory – for those who are overconcerned for the needs of others, friends, relatives or children, continually correcting them and wanting them to conform with their ideas. They are possessive, demanding and can be self-pitying.

Vervain – for those with strong ideas, fixed opinions, those who are always right and wish to teach and convert those around them. They can be over-enthusiastic and overpowering but, during illness, their determination helps them to struggle more than others.

Vine – for strong, capable people, who are self-confident and powerful, certain they are right. They can be dictatorial and overbearing, dominating and directing others with their conviction, even during illness.

Beech – for perfectionists, who need to see more good in all around them and who are easily critical and intolerant. They tend to overlook the positive aspects of other people, over-reacting to minor details and lacking understanding of individual idiosyncracies.

Rock Water – for strictness and self-denial. They shun many of the pleasures in life for fear they will interfere with their work, they drive themselves hard and feel the need to live their lives as an example to others. They want to be strong and fit and will do whatever they believe is necessary to keep them so.

Directions

Take 2 drops of the chosen remedies and place them in a small bottle filled with water and a little brandy if you want to keep it for some time. Take 4 drops of this in a little water, or any convenient way, four times daily or when necessary.

Rescue Remedy

This is the remedy of emergency, for calming emotions during a crisis or trauma. It is made up of Impatiens (for impatience and agitation accompanying stress), Clematis (for unconsciousness or disorientation which can accompany trauma), Rock Rose (for panic, terror and fright), Cherry Plum (for fear of losing mental or physical control) and Star of Bethlehem (for shock, or trauma, either physical or mental).

Directions

Add 4 drops of Rescue Remedy to $\frac{1}{4}$ glass liquid and sip every few minutes or as often as necessary. Hold in the mouth a while before swallowing. Alternatively, place 4 drops under the tongue or in a spoonful of water, *or* rub it on the lips, behind the ears or on the wrists.

APPENDIX 2

FIRST AID CHART

Disorder	First Aid	Herbal Treatments
Sprain and Strains If the pain gets worse after 24 hours call your doctor, as it may mean the underlying bone is broken.	First apply a cold compress or ice packs to help reduce the pain and swelling. Apply a poultice and bandage the area firmly. Change it twice daily.	Use either distilled witch hazel, 1 drop of arnica tincture stirred into a little water, infusion of comfrey, calendula, yarrow or St John's wort, for compress or to freeze into ice cubes. Use comfrey, cabbage leaves, daisies, fresh hyssop or parsley to make a poultice. Use Rescue Remedy for the shock. Rescue Remedy cream or comfrey ointment can also be applied.
Bites and Stings Bee and wasp stings can cause acute allergic reactions in susceptible people. If this occurs call your doctor immediately.	*Bee Stings* Remove a bee sting by pressing it out sideways with your thumbnail rather than pulling it. Press or suck out any poison.	Apply either lavender oil, crushed garlic, distilled witch hazel, infusion of sage, bicarbonate of soda or sliced lemon.
	Wasp Stings If there is nothing else to hand, a little urine can be an excellent first aid remedy.	Apply either cider vinegar, onion, witch hazel, cinnamon or lavender oil, lemon juice or crushed plantain leaves.
	Ant Stings	Raw onion, garlic or cucumber juice will relieve pain when rubbed into the skin.
	Mosquito Bites Try to prevent your child from scratching, as this may introduce infection.	Either lavender, tea tree and rosemary oil, garlic, onion, witch hazel, lemon juice or cider vinegar will relieve irritation. Insect repellent oil can be made from 5 drops of citronella, tea tree, lavender or rosemary oil in 1 teaspoonful (5ml) of base oil. You can also burn dried herbs of rue, rosemary, sage, southernwood, eucalyptus or wormwood in the room.

Disorder	First Aid	Herbal Treatments
Jellyfish Stings		Apply alcohol, papaya juice, vinegar or ammonia.
Splinters Never leave a splinter untreated as it may get septic. If it is large or there is glass, seek medical advice.	First work the area with antiseptic and, if the splinter is easy to get hold of, pull out gently using tweezers. If it is buried under the skin apply a hot poultice or soak affected finger in it for 10–15 minutes. Repeat several times through the day. Once the splinter surfaces, you can pull it out. You may need to use a sterilized needle to ease its passage.	Use a few drops of tincture of either golden seal, calendula or myrrh in a little water to wash the area, make a warm poultice of bread, bran, slippery elm powder, comfrey root or marshmallow, and apply frequently. Apply comfrey, calendula, St John's wort or Rescue Remedy cream and cover. If septic, crush garlic, wrap it in a piece of gauze or cotton and bandage daily. Essential oils of lemon or lavender can also be used.
Sunburn Because sun is very dehydrating, it is important to give plenty of cool water. Extensive sunburn may require medical treatment.	First, cool the area by bathing it with cool water, and take a bath in tepid water. Apply remedies as frequently as required and keep the areas covered when outside, even in the shade.	Apply either fresh cucumber juice, fresh yoghurt, a solution of sodium bicarbonate, aloe vera juice, St John's wort oil or ointment, calendula ointment or an infusion of nettles, chickweed, peppermint, camomile or calendula. Lavender or bergamot oil is also effective – add a few drops to a cool bath. The infusions can also be given internally to cool the system.
Toothache If your child has toothache, visit the dentist.	Herbal remedies can be used in the meantime to relieve the pain.	Apply clove oil on a cotton bud to the area, or tincture of echinacea or myrrh, which have antiseptic properties. Give tea of either hops, valerian, wild lettuce or skullcap.
Travel Sickness This is caused by a disorder of the ear, caused by poor coordination between messages received by the brain from the eyes and from the ears.	Make sure your child looks out of the window and watches the horizon to help balance mechanisms working properly. Do not let him read, encourage interest outside the car, let him sit by the window to get as much fresh air as possible and stay on deck on a boat.	The best remedy is ginger – the fresh root can be chewed, crystallized ginger can be eaten, ginger beer or decoction can be drunk or a few drops of tincture in water can be given. Peppermint and meadowsweet tea are also helpful. Use oils of aniseed, fennel, peppermint or ginger to inhale. If part of the problem is 'nerves', use camomile or skullcap tea.

Disorder	First Aid	Herbal Treatments
Bruises A blow or fall can cause rupture of blood vessels under the skin. If your child bruises easily check his intake of vitamin C and bio-flavonoids. Deficiency can cause fragile blood vessel walls.	Apply a cold compress for $\frac{1}{2}$ hour immediately to contain bruising. Consult your doctor if pain is worse after 24 hours, as it may mean the underlying bone is broken.	Use either witch hazel, or 1 teaspoon (5ml) of calendula, St John's wort, or arnica tincture in $\frac{1}{2}$ pint (300ml) water for compress. Infusions of daisy, yarrow, hyssop or calendula can also be used. Internally 2 drops of Rescue Remedy or 1 drop of arnica tincture stirred into a glass of water will help the shock from the knock or fall. Arnica ointment or Rescue Remedy cream can also be rubbed into the area.
Minor Burns and Scalds If a scald or burn is small and affects only the superficial layer of skin, you can treat it at home. Seek medical advice if pain does not subside with the recommended herbal remedies.	First, immerse the area in cold water for 5–10 minutes or until pain subsides. Raise the affected area slightly to slow blood flow to the area and ease the pain. Do not burst any blisters that form. Seek medical advice if a burn gets more painful or infected.	Apply either neat lavender oil, comfrey ointment, aloe vera juice, St John's wort oil or distilled witch hazel. Infusions of comfrey, calendula, elderflower or plantain can be used as a compress. Repeat frequently to relieve the pain and speed healing. Cover the area loosely with a clean, dry dressing; if it sticks to the skin soak off with warm decoction of echinacea or golden seal.
Minor Cuts and Wounds Probably the worst thing for children is the fall that causes them. If a cut is deep or gaping or there is risk of tetanus, seek medical advice.	Clean the area well with herbal antiseptic to prevent infection and aid healing. If cut is deep, bring the sides together and bind them with surgical tape.	Give Rescue Remedy or 1 drop of arnica stirred into a glass of water immediately; use 4–5 drops of myrrh, golden seal, St John's wort or calendula tincture in a little warm water to wash the area. If very painful, bathe regularly with St John's wort, peppermint or lavender. Cover with a dressing of comfrey, calendula, St John's wort or Rescue Remedy cream.

171

Disorder	First Aid	Herbal Treatments
Fainting and Shock If a child faints and does not regain consciousness, put him in 'recovery position' and call the doctor. Emotional shock is referred to here, not medical shock, which can occur from serious injury and requires urgent medical action.	If your child feels faint, sit him or her down and put the head between the knees to send blood to the head. If already unconscious, lie the child down and raise the legs. Open a window to give fresh air.	Rub rosemary oil into the temples and let the child inhale it from your hands. Give small sips of water or ginger tea to prevent fainting or revive afterwards. For shock there is nothing better than Rescue Remedy or a few drops of arnica tincture stirred into a glass of water. Give teas of rock rose, wild rose flowers, elderflowers or rosemary. For stress that remains give camomile, lemon balm or skullcap, and give Rescue Remedy four times daily.
Nosebleeds If they occur after a blow to the head they can be a sign of fracture, seek medical help immediately. If they occur frequently consult doctor.	Hold the nostrils firmly together and lie the child down for a few minutes until the bleeding stops. Do not let the child blow the nose or sniff as this could dislodge the clot and start bleeding again. Vitamin C and bioflavonoids will help strengthen capillary walls and help prevent frequent nosebleeds.	Apply a cold compress of distilled witch hazel, St John's wort, calendula or yarrow tincture to the back of the neck and hold cotton wool soaked in one of these to the nose. Alternatively, a few drops of cypress oil may be inhaled or applied to the nose.
Chilblains These are related to poor circulation, and aggravated by tight shoes, poor diet and lack of exercise.	Encourage the child to take plenty of exercise and wear warm clothes.	Dust the feet with a pinch of cayenne pepper mixed with talc or arrowroot powder before putting on socks or tights. Give hot hand and foot baths of ginger and cinnamon. Give garlic and ginger tea internally. Apply friar's balsam neat to unbroken chilblains. Garlic oil, tincture of myrrh, nettle juice, onion juice and salt water are also helpful.

APPENDIX 3

DIET CHART

Sources	Function	Supplements
Protein First class: meat, poultry, fish, eggs, milk, soya products. Second class: nuts and seeds, beans and pulses, grains. Two out of the three groups must be combined together in the same meal to make a first class protein equivalent.	For the basic building blocks of all body tissues, many important hormones and antibodies.	Ample supply is necessary, particularly in childhood, adolescence, pregnancy and lactation.
Fats *Essential Fatty Acids*: Seeds, nuts, pulses, beans, unrefined vegetable oils, oily fish, fish liver oils.	Vital to normal development of nervous and immune systems. They form the major structural part of the cell wall in every cell in the body. Necessary for absorption of trace elements and fat-soluble vitamins A, E, D and K. Involved in synthesis of adrenal and sex hormones and maintenance of healthy bacterial population of the gut, for healthy skin and circulation.	Useful in disturbances of ovulation and menstruation; increased blood cholesterol levels, atherosclerosis, hypertension and multiple sclerosis; lowered immunity and nervous problems. Cod liver oil, 1 tablespoonful (20ml) daily and evening primrose oil, 500mg daily, are useful sources.
Saturated Fats: Dairy produce, meats, processed fats, refined oils.	Provide concentrated energy, provide insulation and protection. Should be kept to a minimum as excessive amounts predispose to cardio-vascular problems, obesity and many other problems.	

Sources	Function	Supplements
Carbohydrates		
Whole grains, fruits, vegetables, nuts, seeds, pulses, beans.	Complex carbohydrates help reduce the risk of cardio-vascular disease. The indigestible fibre is essential to healthy bowel function and protects against bowel disease, gall stones and reduces cholesterol levels. Contain nutrients to aid digestion and supply energy.	
Vitamins		
Vitamin A (fat soluble) Fish oils, milk produce, (organic) liver, egg yolk, carrots. Carotene is a precursor of Vitamin A, found in green, yellow and orange vegetables, and orange and yellow fruits.	Builds resistance to infections, promotes growth, healthy hair, teeth, skin and gums, and helps repair tissues. Necessary for healthy eyes, bone formation, digestion, red and white blood cell production, and foundation of hormones involved with reproduction and lactation.	To prevent infections and help resolve acute respiratory infections. To help skin conditions such as acne, boils and infections such as impetigo. Good for weak eyes, and hyperthyroidism. Take in cod liver oil, 1 tablespoon (20ml) daily.
Vitamin B1 (thiamin, water soluble) Whole grains, oatmeal, (organic) liver, legumes, yeast, milk, nuts, lentils, seeds and eggs.	Essential for metabolism of carbohydrates, to glucose or fat, and for energy production.	Useful for those recovering from infections or suffering emotional problems. Can relieve fatigue headaches, neuralgia, depression, irritability, poor memory or sensitivity to cold and pain. 10–50mg daily in B-complex or brewer's yeast.
Vitamin B2 (riboflavin) Milk, cheese, butter, yoghurt, cereals, meat, brewer's yeast, wheatgerm, green leaf vegetables, beans, peas and eggs.	Involved with formation of liver enzymes and use of oxygen in energy metabolism of carbohydrates, fats and proteins stored in the liver.	Requirements are increased in times of growth (childhood), pregnancy and lactation and with a high-protein diet. Useful for sore tongue and lips, sensitivity to light, skin problems, 10–20mg daily in B-complex or brewer's yeast.

Sources	Function	Supplements
Vitamin B3 (nicotinic acid/ niacin) Whole grains, milk produce, meat, fish, brewer's yeast, green vegetables, nuts and eggs.	Involved with formation of enzymes necessary for carbohydrate metabolism. Affects cholesterol metabolism and helps reduce blood fats.	Deficiency is linked to high alcohol consumption and low protein intake. May be helpful for skin problems, diarrhoea, mouth ulcers, sore tongue, poor memory, depression, tension and anxiety. Helps protect against the effects of herbicides and pesticides. 50mg daily in B-complex or brewer's yeast.
Vitamin B5 (pantothenic acid) Cow's milk, breast milk, eggs, cereals, meat, brewer's yeast, green vegetables and mushrooms.	Involved with metabolism of carbohydrates, fats and amino acids. The adrenal glands depend on it to function normally and to produce adequate adrenal hormones. Helps the immune system.	Needs are increased during pregnancy, lactation, illness, injury, healing and emotional stress. Useful for insomnia, depression, cramps, digestive disturbances, nausea and vomiting, burning feet, numbness and tingling, arthritis and gout. 5–10mg daily in B-complex.
Vitamin B6 (pyridoxine) Fish, meat, egg yolk, whole grains, nuts and seeds, green vegetables, brewer's yeast, bananas, avocados, molasses and mushrooms.	Involved in metabolism of proteins and amino acids, sugars and fatty acids, and some minerals. Aids manufacture of red blood cells, antibodies, hormones and enzymes.	For prevention of cardiovascular disease, skin disease, inflammatory conditions and immune problems. Needs are increased by high protein intake, as in pregnancy and lactation, in those who smoke and drink, by taking drugs and by food additives and stress. 5–10mg daily to correct deficiencies.
Vitamin B12 (cyano-cobalamin) Meat, liver, kidneys, fish, eggs, milk produce, bean sprouts. Also manufactured by intestinal bacteria.	For normal development of red blood cells, for iron metabolism and for a healthy nervous system.	For pernicious anaemia, symptoms linked to the nervous system, including numbness and tingling in hands and feet, neuritis and clumsiness. Also menstrual irregularities, back pain, tiredness, bowel problems and skin disorder. 3–4mg in B-complex daily.
Folic acid Brewer's yeast, green vegetables, eggs, whole grains, meat, nuts and milk.	For red blood cell formation in bone marrow. For metabolism of sugar, amino acids and manufacture of antibodies. Crucial to normal function of the nervous system and for production of RNA and DNA, which determine hereditary patterns.	Needs are increased during pregnancy, lactation, growth and stress, by the pill, alcohol and some drugs. 400–800mg daily for anaemia, fatigue, dizziness, depression, susceptibility to infection, sore tongue and cracks at corners of mouth.

Sources	Function	Supplements
Vitamin C Fresh fruit and vegetables, potatoes, leafy herbs and berries.	Vital for healthy skin, bones and muscles, as it is involved with collagen production. Also for healing and protection from the effects of viruses, toxins, drugs, allergies and foreign bodies. Necessary for cholesterol metabolism and production of cortisol by the adrenals. Enhances resistance and iron absorption, and is an effective anti-oxidant.	Helps reduce effects of toxic metals, needs increase during stress, injury, surgery, infection, drug therapy, smoking and drinking. For poor resistance, weakness and fatigue, capillary fragility, tender muscles and joints. 500–1000mg daily.
Vitamin D Milk produce, eggs, fatty fish, fish oil. Synthesized in the skin from sunlight.	Vital for normal calcium formation and growth and health of bones and teeth. Increases absorption of calcium and phosphates from diet.	For hot flushes, night sweats, bone fragility, tooth decay, cramp, irritability and depression. Take in cod liver oil, 1 dessertspoonful (12ml) daily.
Vitamin E Nuts and seeds, eggs, milk produce, whole grains, wheat germ, unrefined oils, leafy vegetables, avocados, seaweeds, soya beans, breast milk.	For metabolism of essential fatty acids, absorption of iron, for red blood cell manufacture; antioxidant, protects the circulatory system and cells, and slows the aging process. Increases fertility and protects against development of foetal abnormalities and miscarriage.	To speed healing of wounds for vascular problems – varicose veins, phlebitis – to prevent anaemia, heart diseases, strokes, muscle degeneration and premature aging. For menopausal flushes 200–400iu daily. *NB* Avoid if on anti-coagulants or if you have high blood pressure, diabetes or hyperthyroidism, or toxaemia of pregnancy; separate iron from Vitamin E supplements by 8 hours.
Vitamin K Green vegetables, milk products, molasses, apricots, whole grains, cod liver oil, garlic, sunflower oil. Synthesized in the intestines.	For production of blood clotting factors, notably prothrombin.	
Minerals and Trace Elements		
Sodium Most vegetables, salt.	Vital for maintenance of fluid balance and blood pressure and normal nerve and muscle function.	Needs increased by excessive sweating, vigorous exercise, saunas; for nausea, vomiting, dizziness, cramps, tiredness, resulting from this.

Sources	Function	Supplements
Calcium Milk produce, green vegetables, eggs, nuts, seeds, dried fruit, soya beans, bony fish, cereals.	For healthy bones and teeth, normal function of heart muscle, blood clotting mechanisms, condition of nerve impulses and muscle function.	Enhances resistance to infection and allergies by its effect on the immune system. For muscle pain, cramps, PMT, period pains, growing pains, osteoporosis, osteomalacia, back pain, insomnia, tension, irritability, indigestion and constipation. 400–500mg daily.
Iron Egg yolk, liver, meat, molasses, soya beans, whole grains, green vegetables, fish, dried fruits, cocoa and wine.	Used in production of haemoglobin, vital for transport of oxygen in the blood. Important to energy production and cellular respiration, promotes growth and protein.	For anaemia, weakness, headaches, palpitations, depression and poor memory; needs increase during pregnancy, lactation, growth and repair. 10–20mg daily.
Magnesium Green vegetables, nuts, seeds, whole grains, milk produce, eggs, seafoods, 'hard' water.	For energy production, protein metabolism, manufacture of enzymes, nerve and muscle function, bone and teeth formation.	For tension and irritability. Tremors and twitches, spasms and convulsions, insomnia, leg and foot cramps, apathy, depression, poor memory, hyperactivity and muscle weakness. Needs increased in diarrhoea, excessive urination, alcoholism and pregnancy. 300–400mg daily.
Phosphorus Whole grains, seeds, nuts, meat, fish, eggs.	Vital for healthy bone formation and heart and kidney function. Important for nerve conduction and vitamin metabolism.	
Potassium Fresh fruit and vegetables, whole grains, nuts, soya beans, milk, seafood.	For nerve conduction and muscle function, to regulate acid/alkali balance of blood, and water balance in the blood.	Needs increased when using diuretics. For muscle weakness, cramps, fatigue, insomnia, low blood sugar, constipation. Take in salt substitutes.
Copper Green vegetables, liver, seafoods, whole grains.	For formation of myelin sheath around nerves, iron formation, enzyme production, development of brain, bones and, with B6, of connective tissue. Acts as an antioxidant. Essential for use of vitamin C.	Needs increased in pregnancy, kidney disease, hypertension, diets high in milk produce, saturated fats and sugar. For raised cholesterol levels and other cardiovascular problems. 2–5mg daily.

Sources	Function	Supplements
Zinc Oysters, herrings, yeast, liver, egg, beef, peas, seeds, fruit and vegetables, nuts, poultry, shellfish.	A component of about 90 enzymes. For protein metabolism, helps prevent free-radical damage of the eyes, prostate, seminal fluid and sperm. For normal immune function and hormone production and healthy bones and joints. Required for release of vitamin A from liver stores.	For prevention or treatment of infection allergies or auto-immune disease. Helps wound healing. Needs increased by infections, diabetes, liver disease, smoking, alcohol, drugs, strenuous exercise, 'hard' water and diets high in fibre. For skin problems, joint pain, menstrual irregularities, lack of taste and smell, coeliac disease, stomach, ulcers, ulcerative colitis, hyperactivity and Crohn's disease. 15mg daily.
Cobalt Brewer's yeast, fruit and vegetables, whole grains, nuts.	A component of vitamin B12. Enhances copper absorption and magnesium and sugar metabolism.	
Manganese Green vegetables, seeds, whole grains, pulses, brewer's yeast, eggs, fruits, tea.	Important for energy metabolism, healthy bones, thyroid function and the nervous and reproductive systems.	To soothe histamine-mediated allergic reactions, such as hay fever and urticaria. For poor growth, anaemia, nervous disorders, poor maternal instinct and learning difficulties. 10–30mg daily of manganese chloride.
Iodine Vegetables grown on iodine-rich soils, fruits, seafoods, garlic, parsley, iodized salt.	Vital to production of thyroid hormones, responsible for regulating metabolism and physical and mental development.	To help eliminate poisons such as radiation and heavy metals. For decreased thyroid production with fatigue, susceptibility to cold, low libido, low blood pressure, weight gain and raised blood cholesterol. In kelp or iodized salt.
Chromium Fruit and vegetables, meat, molasses, whole grains, wheatgerm, brewer's yeast, organic foods.	Vital for fat and carbohydrate metabolism, and production of energy.	For diabetes as it potentiates insulin. Enhances growth and longevity. For high blood pressure and arteriosclerosis. Take in brewer's yeast.
Selenium Garlic, whole grains, eggs, meat, brewer's yeast.	Antioxidant, vital for normal liver function, connective tissue and formation of sex hormones.	Combines with toxic metals and helps to remove them from the body. For infertility, allergies, joint pains, muscle weakness. May protect against cancer and cataracts and heart disease. *NB* Supplementation only under advice from your practitioner except when taken in kelp or brewer's yeast.

APPENDIX 4

HERBAL SUPPLIERS

Midsummer Herbs,
Nether Westcote, near Kingham,
Oxon OX7 6SD (tel: 0993 830419)

Mayway Herbs
34 Greek Street,
London W1 (tel: 071–494–3612)

Potters Herbal Supplies Ltd,
Leyland Mill Lane, Wigan,
Lancashire WN1 2SB (tel: 0942 34761)

Brome & Schimmer Ltd,
5 Bridge Road Estate, Romsey,
Hampshire SO5 0HR (tel: 0794 515595)

Pierce Arnold & Son,
Pollard Road, Morden,
Surrey SM4 6EG (tel: 081-647 5330)

G. Baldwin & Co.,
171–173 Walworth Road,
London SE17 1RW (tel: 071-703 5550)

Neals Yard Apothecary,
2 Neals Yard, Covent Garden,
London WC2H 9DP

Bach Flower Remedies,
from Dr Edward Bach Centre,
Mount Vernon, Sotwell, Wallingford,
Oxon OX10 0PZ

Cathay of Bournemouth Ltd,
32 Cleveland Road,
Bournemouth, Dorset

Culpeper Ltd,
21 Bruton Street, Berkeley Square,
London W1X 7OA

Gerard House Ltd,
736 Christchurch Road,
Bournemouth, Dorset

Napier & Sons,
18 Nicholson Street, Edinburgh EH8 9DJ

APPENDIX 5

USEFUL ADDRESSES

Women's Health Information Centre,
52 Featherstone Street, London EC1

British Association for Counselling,
37a Sheep Street, Rugby CV21 3BX

British Association of Psychotherapists,
121 Hendon Lane, London N3 3PR

Westminster Pastoral Foundation,
23 Kensington Square, London W8

National Childbirth Trust,
Alexandra House, Oldham Terrace, Acton,
London W3 6NH

Active Birth Centre,
55 Dartmouth Park Road,
London NW5

Research Council for Complementary
Medicine,
Suite 1, 19a Cavendish Square,
London W1

National Institute of Medical Herbalists,
9 Palace Gate, Exeter, Devon

The Herb Society,
77 Great Peter Street, London SW1

Dr Edward Bach Centre,
Mount Vernon, Sotwell, Wallingford,
Oxon OX10 0PZ

School of Meditation,
158 Holland Park Avenue, London W11

Clinical Theology Association,
St Mary's House, Church Westcote,
near Kingham, Oxford.

REFERENCES

INTRODUCTION

1. Fulder, S. and Munro, R., *Lancet*, 2, pp. 542–5, 1985
2. Griggs, Barbara, *Green Pharmacy* Norman & Hobhouse, 1981
3. McCleb, Rob, *Herbalgram*, 13, pp. 12–13, Society for Econ Bot, Symposium on the Investigation of Folk Medicine, 1987
4. *Herbalgram*, 20, spring 1989

CHAPTER 2

1. Griggs, Barbara, *Green Pharmacy*, Norman & Hobhouse, 1981
2. Vogel, V.J., *Indian Herbal Medicine*, Oklahoma Press, 1970
3. Vogel, ibid.

CHAPTER 5

1. Ainsworth and Weber, Spitz, R., *The First Year of Life*, International University Press, New York, 1965
2. Stanway, P., *Green Babies*, Century, London, 1990
3. *Nutritional Health*, 4, p. 8, 1985
4. Chilton Pearce, *Nutrition and Health*, vol. 1, no 3 and 4

5. Stanway, P., op. cit.
6. For a list of drugs and their effects see Stanway, P., op. cit.
7. Airola, P., *1977 Environmental Defense Fund Study*, Everywoman's Book, Health Plus Publishers, Phoenix, Arizona, 1979

CHAPTER 8

1. Shiller, G., *Childhood Illness*, Unwin, 1974, 1979
2. Felder, S., 'How to Survive Medical Treatment', D.T.K. *Lancet*, 2, p. 1174, 1975
3. Peters, T. and Bjarnason, I., in *Food and the Gut*, Balliere Tindall, 1985
4. Hildenbrand, G.J., *Alternative Medicine*, 16–23 February 1986
5. Stanway, A., *Natural Family Doctor*, Gaia, 1987, p. 114
6. Weiss, R.F., *Herbal Medicine*, Beaconsfield, Arcanum 1988
7. Weiss, R.F., op. cit.

CHAPTER 9

1. Weiss, R.F., op. cit.
2. Davis, S. and Stewart, A., *Nutritional Medicine*, Pan Books Ltd, London, 1987

BIBLIOGRAPHY

Airola, P., *Every Woman's Book*, Health Plus Publishers, Phoenix, Arizona, 1979

Balaskas, J., *Natural Pregnancy*, Sidgwick & Jackson Ltd, London, 1990

Ballantine, R., *Diet and Nutrition*, Himalayan International Institute, Honesdale, Pennsylvania, 1978

Campion, K., *A Woman's Herbal*, Century, London, 1987

Campion, K., *The Family Medical Herbal*, Dorling Kindersley Ltd, London, 1988

Chancellor, P., *Handbook of Bach Flower Remedies*, Keats Publishing Inc., Connecticut, 1980 and The C.W. Daniel Company Ltd, Saffron Waldon, Essex, 1985

Charles, R., *Mind, Body and Immunity*, Methuen, London, 1990

Davis, S. and Stewart, A., *Nutritional Medicine*, Pan Books Ltd, London, 1987

de Bairacli Levy, Juliette, *The Illustrated Herbal Handbook*, Faber & Faber Ltd, London, 1974

de Bairacli Levy, Juliette, *Natural Rearing of Children*, Faber & Faber Ltd, London, 1970

Elkington, J., *The Poisoned Womb*, Penguin Books Ltd, Harmondsworth, Middlesex, 1986

Galland, L., *Superimmunity for Kids*, Bloomsbury Publishing Ltd, London, 1989

Grieve, M., *A Modern Herbal*, Penguin Books Ltd, Harmondsworth, Middlesex, 1976

Griggs, Barbara, *Green Pharmacy*, Norman & Hobhouse, 1981

Lovelock, James, *Gaia: A New Look at Life on Earth*, Oxford University Press, 1979

Mabey, R. and McIntyre, M., *The Complete New Herbal*, Elm Tree Books, London, 1988

McIntyre, A., *Herbs for Pregnancy and Childbirth*, Sheldon Press Ltd, London, 1988

McIntyre, M., *Herbal Medicine for Everyone*, Penguin Books Ltd, Harmondsworth, Middlesex, 1988

National Childbirth Trust, *Pregnancy and Parenthood*, Oxford University Press, 1985

Parvati, Jeannine, *Hygieia*, Wildwood House Ltd, Aldershot, Hampshire, 1978

Philips, A. and Rakusen, J., *Our Bodies, Ourselves*, Penguin Books Ltd, Harmondsworth, Middlesex, 1978

Phillips, D., *New Dimensions in Health*, Angus & Robertson, London, 1977

Scheffer, M., *Bach Flower Therapy*, Thorsons Publishers Ltd, Wellingborough, 1986

Sheldrake, Rupert, *A New Science of Life*, Blond & Briggs, London, 1988

Schiller, J., *Childhood Illness*, Unwin Hyman Ltd, London, 1979

Scott, Julian, *Natural Medicine for Children*, Unwin Hyman Ltd, London, 1990

Stanway, P., *Green Babies*, Century, London, 1990

Vogel, V.J., *American Indian Medicine*, Oklahoma Press, 1970

Weiss, R.F., *Herbal Medicine*, Beaconsfield Publishers, Arcanum, 1988

Worwood, V., *The Fragrant Pharmacy*, Macmillan, London, 1990

GENERAL INDEX

travel sickness 137, 170
trigeminal neuralgia 28

ulcerative colitis 36, 67, 69
umbilical cord, dressing 46
urethritis 23
urinary infections 36, 83,
    142, 155–6
urinary system 19, 20, 23,
    35, 154–7
urticaria *see* hives

vaginal secretions 19
varicose veins 27, 28, 35
verrucae 150–1

vital force 13–14, 18, 80, 86,
    89
vitamins 19, 21, 37, 62–63,
    66, 69, 71, 72, 73, 74, 77,
    96, 99, 104, 112, 115,
    119, 122, 125, 126, 127,
    128, 129, 138, 144, 145,
    148, 150, 151, 152, 162,
    163, 174–6
volatile oils 19–20, 23
vomiting 50–1, 80, 81, 82,
    107, 114, 116, 131–3,
    134, 136, 137, 138, 142,
    143, 155, 161

warts 150–1
weaning 43
whooping cough 108,
    113–16
wind 125, 142, 143
World Health
    Organization 9, 17
worms 124, 134, 140–1

zinc 63, 69, 71, 73, 96, 126,
    127, 128, 145, 178

INDEX OF HERBS